TANTRA WITHOUT TEARS

TANTRA WITHOUT TEARS

by
Christopher S. Hyatt, Ph.D.
&
S. Jason Black

NEW FALCON PUBLICATIONS
TEMPE, ARIZONA, U.S.A.

International Standard Book Number: 1-56184-060-2
Library of Congress Catalog Card Number: 96-67336

First Edition 1999

Cover Art by Nancy Wasserman

The paper used in this publication meets the minimum requirements of the American National Standard for Permanence of Paper for Printed Library Materials Z39.48-1984

Address all inquiries to:
NEW FALCON PUBLICATIONS
PMB 277
1739 East Broadway Road #1
Tempe, AZ 85282 U.S.A.
(or)
PMB 286
320 East Charleston Blvd. • Suite 204
Las Vegas, NV 89104 U.S.A.

website: http://www.newfalcon.com
email: info@newfalcon.com

Table of Contents

Introduction

For the Western Mind this is the only Book on Tantra you will ever need.

A bold statement?

Maybe. However, the idea behind this book is simple.

It is power.

It is Kundalini, dressed in Western clothes.

It describes experiences and techniques which allow you to glimpse beyond ordinary day-to-day reality, into a world of marvels and horrors.

This book is the result of these marvels and horrors. In fact, it was not written as a traditional book at all, but was spontaneously dictated in altered states of consciousness inspired as were many Esoteric books of the past.

Thus, this book is a spontaneous outpouring of our own refusal to accept how books such as this must be done.

We responded to questions by speaking into a tape recorder. From the transcription we organized and edited the book to retain its natural and mysterious quality.

In this sense this book is somewhat experimental. The book is an extended conversation or dialogue among individuals—as indeed were many of the original Tantras.

Over the years we have had questions asked us about Tantra and Magick. Many of these came from readers of our other jointly written books while others came from reading Dr. Hyatt's two books on Western Tantra.

As Westerners who practice Magick and Tantra, some of our responses to the questions are designed to penetrate the Western Mind Set.

Thus, do not expect a series of foreign words (some might call it 'hindu babble') strung together as an answer to a question. To us, such approaches are nothing more than the refusal to answer the question by making the simple complex—for the benefit of the writer's ego.

It would be ridiculous for us to answer questions by employing esoteric Eastern concepts. If we did, this book would be of little use for the Western practitioner.

We do not pretend to be experts in the phraseology, language, culture, etc. of the Eastern path. *What we are expert in is the utilization of their techniques to accomplish the desired ends.*

In many instances we will deliberately use Western methods and symbols as they are easier for the Western collective unconscious to assimilate and integrate.

Two other books we have written—*Pacts With the Devil* (1993) and *Urban Voodoo* (1995), both New Falcon Publications—have this theme in common: practical results based on experience and theoretical knowledge.

This book will give you the understanding and ability to use certain symbols, sounds and images that you will find in more conventional and classical texts.

In other words, as well as an instructional text, it is also a jumping off point for those who wish to pursue the original Eastern material at another time.

This book tells you how to achieve and utilize power to meet your own needs and suit your own ends.

It is not about *common* notions of harmony or angels or anything like that. It is not sweet-and-light and is full of real-world experiences which reflect the workings of Tantric philosophy and practice.

By the way, the title of this book was suggested by analogy to Aleister Crowley's *Magick Without Tears* (New Falcon Publications) which consists of a series of questions and answers on Western mysticism. We had received many questions stimulated by our other works and which we felt required answers. So we decided to steal Crowley's approach to answering these questions. So, in this sense, this book is written by our many readers to whom we give eternal thanks.

1

Why is the subject of Tantra so confusing?

Tantra has been a confusing issue for most Westerners. Most of us don't know what it really is. And if you sit down and read a typical book about Tantra you are often overwhelmed by five or ten words in a row for which the student has no reference or understanding. Not only is there a problem of pronunciation and memorization, there is also a problem of translation.

Many of the available Western versions of the original Eastern texts try to remain faithful to the original material but at the cost of incomprehensible terminology, mistakes of translation, proliferation of unsupported concepts and unavoidable confusions of cultural context.

So the message of *Tantra Without Tears* is to remove some of the misery and pain that accompany the study of this particular topic. Some of the questions and answers in this work come from letters that were written to us from students asking questions on Tantra or 'Sex Magick.'

2

What does the word Tantra mean?

The word 'Tantra' itself is a good example of things that don't have a terribly clear meaning even in their native land. The Tantras themselves are a group of writings that are considered sacred and have various degrees of complexity. Some of them are high poetry, like the *Tantra of the Great Liberation.*

Others are only a few pages long, are rather crudely written, and are really very little different than some European Grimoires.

The word *Tantra,* from our point of view, broadly indicates *action.*

It indicates unity between theory and practice.

The image of a loom has been used frequently with Tantra being the shuttle that guides the threads to create an entire cloth in much the same way as the word Yoga has been compared with a yoke to which oxen have been attached to pull a cart.

3

What is the place of religious dogma in Tantra?

From the point of view of Tantra, dogma itself is essentially useless (or, if you would, a prop for a new student) and any form of dogma can be disregarded once it has ceased to be useful. However, it is important to keep in mind that dogma helps some people begin and continue on a path until they are ready to drop the dogma. Most people 'practice' dogma and not Tantra or Magick.

4

What is the basic goal of Tantra?

The thing that shocks most Westerners (and a great many orthodox Hindus) about Tantra is the fact that the *highest good* is considered to be the development of the aspirant *as he defines it* without the cloak of external morality.

From a Tantric point of view, whatever one does, acceptable by society or not, is simply the means to the same end—self-development.

It should be remembered that antinomianism (deliberate renunciation of social and religious restrictions) in Tantra—as in so many secret doctrines—is fundamental.

In this sense most American authors on Tantra would vigorously disagree as their training and public persona are conventional. Many of these people come from an academic background.

As for ourselves, Dr. Hyatt has an extensive background in real world psychotherapy (that is, he worked with real patients, as compared to just lecturing to students). He has held licenses as a clinical psychologist and as a marriage and family therapist and has been a fellow in a number of organizations and so on and so forth. He has an extensive background in classical psychotherapy as well as the more unusual forms of psychotherapy[1].

Jason Black has a background in the arts, worked for nearly a decade in 'the business' in Hollywood, and acted as psychic advisor during this period to a number of film professionals.

---

[1] Please note that Dr. Hyatt has retired from his work as a psychotherapist. Nor is he available to provide referals to other therapists.

From different directions, we have, combined, nearly a half-century of experience in the practice of various Occult and Yogic techniques.

The essential problem now as always is the unconscious tendency to view alien philosophy through the lens of the ingrained and familiar culture. In the West, Judeo-Christian values dominate our thinking and perceptions, act as values of faith and are anti-empirical.

All forms of Yoga, whether Tantra or otherwise, demand empirical results not faith.

In this sense these practices are closer to Western Science.

From the monotheistic point of view, Tantrism—whether Buddhist or Hindu—is dangerous and diabolical even as a philosophy.

Engaging in any practice devoted to self-determinism may put you beyond the scope of society. This should be kept in mind as you gain more power, as one of the first mistakes of any serious student is talking about his most secret goals. What may seem harmless to you may be a panic trigger to someone else.

5

How many types of Tantra are there?

Although there are 'hundreds' of sects there are, broadly speaking, two schools of thought: the Hindu Tantras which are theistic and come primarily from Bengal in India and Tibetan which, being Buddhist, doesn't involve the worship of gods although it does acknowledge Spiritual Beings.

To make things clearer for the Western Reader, many Tibetan Buddhists may acknowledge the existence of beings called gods, but do not deem them worthy of worship and in some cases even worthy of interest.

Early Taoism in China also shares many of these qualities.

6

What is the history of Tantra?

No comprehensive history of Tantra has been written. The origin of the techniques stretches back to pre-historic Shamanism.

Recorded history is basically this: according to historians the original Tantras were probably Buddhist and originated in India. However, eventually Buddhism faded from India for a variety of reasons; the primary cause was the Islamic invasion of India which destroyed a great deal of Tantric heritage and thousands and thousands of books.

When the influence of the Islamic empire in India faded, what recovered was classical Hinduism and not Buddhism. Buddhism essentially faded from the place where Buddha himself lived moving to China and then to Japan.

After this the Tantric techniques and philosophy still existed but were kept secret because of their shocking nature. You can imagine how shocked the Islamic invaders were when they learned about the practices that were going on because the only person more uptight about sex than a Jew or a Christian is a Moslem.

As a result, what was once a widespread, recognized cult in India became hidden and esoteric. And this is what makes the Hindu Tantras particularly useful. Being secret, they were no longer subject to public opinion and thus were more direct. However, the Hindu Tantras, because of the destructive effects of history, are also very confused.

To eliminate some of the confusion we've gone to the Buddhist Tantras of Tibet and there the essential purity of the original doctrine has been preserved to a great degree.

The only exception being the doctrines regarding sex and morality.

The ruling powers of Tibet at a relatively early period in their history after their contact with India decided that Tantric Buddhism was to be the national religion.

They poured all their resources, intellectual and financial, into creating universities and libraries.

It remained a powerful esoteric influence with authority figures, traditions, even families involved in it going back generations and even centuries. The literature is rich—even richer than we can imagine since only a certain portion of it has ever been translated into English.

This provides ground for a fully realized tradition and fully realized practice. This, combined with the fact that doctors and hospitals in the East have no problem dealing with Kundalini phenomena provides something of a safety net for the practitioner.

In Tibet, Tantra has been the government since the 7th century. Entire universities were devoted to it and, like any large organization, they have ways of dealing with people with various talents—lay talent, high talent and genius. And the people at the top, as within any hierarchy were more or less separated from the general membership.

For the purposes of this book we agree with the Buddhists that most of, if not all of the concepts of the self that we have—the idea of a soul or as the Hindus would put it the "Atman"—is delusion, a convenient construct for the control of the masses and for an "understanding" of the Universe.

7

What do Buddhists mean by Illusion?

When we use the words "illusion" and "delusion" throughout this book, we are not talking about "hallucination."

When Buddhists talk about illusion they are not talking about something that isn't there. They are talking about the structure of language to describe and to define what exists or not. They are saying we use definitions to define things which, by their nature, can't be defined.

The definition of "definition" is limitation. As such, when we speak of something which, in reality, is process, it appears that we talking about it as a thing. This we call "thinging-It." It is difficult for language to convey the thingness of something and, at the same time, its non-thingness.

Thinging-It is a process that we run into over and over again, usually beginning with Westerners' first exposure to Buddhism: they are looking for clear nouns, verbs and predicates. Sadly, this often results in rejection out-of-hand (unless, of course, they are a Christian Scientist, in which case the mistake takes a different and more perverse turn).

Another concept that the Buddhists use (which can take years to figure out unaided) is that of the "void." When you read about the void in an English translation you normally think it means, "there is nothing there." That's not what it means at all. The void refers to the fact that "mind" cannot be separated from "matter" and that neither mind nor matter can be defined in Western terms; yet words must be used to point to the experience.

8

Do matter and mind exist?

Whatever matter "is" cannot be separated from whatever mind "is." These are just terms to note certain differences, but not Ultimate categories. Again, we run into the problem of discrete categories and, unlike Tibetans, do not assume an Ultimate form of interconnectedness.

Nothing can be stated to exist in a purely "physical" state as we understand it and nothing "not" to exist in this state, but under normal states of consciousness we must act *as if* they are completely different. Which is why, when you deal with Tibetan Buddhism and Tibetan Tantra, you have a lot of images to separate and integrate at will the various planes and forces.

9

If Tantra is not a Religion, why so many Gods and Demons?

There are a great many demons and Bodhisattvas who were never real people in the sense a Westerner would understand it but are considered to be real on their own level. One reason for the multiple "God" formula is similar to practices found in both Zen and Kabbalah: the collapse of all differences—which is often termed "enlightenment"—only to be followed by the re-affirmation of all differences which is *also* termed enlightenment.

To deal or cope with a God or Demon, whether internal or external, doesn't necessarily mean that it must be worshipped.

It is our delusion in the West, that Gods "must" be worshipped.

These principles are difficult to convey in language because they defy it since language is both process and category and neither. Language has its own existence and thus its own prejudices.

10

*What is the Reality of our images that appear to us
more or less spontaneously?*

Translators have tended to make Tantric experiences
seem as though they were *merely* a psychological construct
generated by one's mental activity. This is like using the
language and principles of physics to describe psychological activity. It is reductionism of the unknown to the pre-
tended known.

Some images have "physical structure" just as "real" as a
person sitting across the room. But others have a quality to
them that is very hard to put your finger on. They may be
products of mind but, if they are, they're not the products of
any sort of rational thought.

They appear to be images of living people. Sometimes
they come to teach us things.

On some occasions they have accomplished almost
miraculous physical effects on physical bodies and sur-
roundings but at the same time this does not necessarily
lead to the conclusion that they are literally people or
spirits.

On the other hand, we have made it clear in previous
books that after almost fifty years of serious practice of
ceremonial Magick we believe in spirits as much as we
believe in people (or as little). So, if we can get past these
confusions the practitioner will be able to understand, and
hopefully deal with, some of the things that are inevitably
going to happen to him in the course of meditation and in
the course of the quasi-magical processes that are involved
in Tantra.

11

What about God?

We agree with the Buddhists that it is fruitless to start
talking about God. This is the downfall of most occult
practices. It becomes religion.

Interestingly, it becomes religion mostly in the Christian
sense. The idea of creator-gods (or God) is a question the
Buddha himself flatly stated was intellectually a waste of
time. It's an absurd question. If something appears to us
and claims to be a God and satisfies us with the proper I.D.,
then we might buy it.

However, generally speaking, in both Hindu and Buddhist Tantra, these things are only paid attention to if they
are useful or make themselves noted in ways which can't
be ignored.

We can think of one example of the possible utility of a
God-image. In Gopi Krishna's account of his Kundalini
experience which he worked up to for a number of years,
(and Krishna, whom you might not be familiar with, was a
Hindu Tantric) he was practicing Kundalini Yoga without
visualizing anything but the force rising up his spine to the
top of his head.

One morning the Kundalini rose for the first time. It created such great physical and psychological problems that it
took him years to control these difficulties. From our own
experience we can say that Kundalini happens when it is
least expected and if it is an exclusively pleasant experience
you are very lucky.

Another Hindu Tantric made a remark about Gopi Krishna's experience saying that, if he had visualized a deity
during this experience, he would not have had a painful

result. This is simply an assertion on his part as far as we know but he may be right. So bear in mind that the symbols used are often anthropomorphic and this may be an efficient safety valve.

12

Is Tantra primarily philosophy or Yoga?

Tantra is a body of technique and physical practice—and we want to emphasize *physical* practice—combined with certain metaphysical assumptions about the world that are in themselves provable from personal experience but not necessarily from rigorous scientific testing.

They do not involve moral dogma except in their esoteric sense, they do not involve personal limitations, nor do they involve issues of right and wrong apart from the progress of the aspirant.

Basically Tantra is a body of practice combined with a body of theory aimed at the ultimate development of the practitioner into his highest form. You can carry this methodology in any direction you like, whether you are dealing with the concepts of life after death, or personal power in the physical world.

13

If the nature of reality is indeterminate, how do we judge our experiences?

You have no choice, you will judge them.

As we face the concepts of illusion or hallucination or delusion we must always keep in mind that no matter what we experience we experience it *through* (and we emphasize the word "through") a particular set of organs and a particular type of brain.

This does *not* mean that what you experience is not "real" or does not have some form of spiritual or energetic base (although many would assert that precisely because you experience something means that it does not exist at all). It *does* mean that you do not see or experience the entity or force as it exists independent of the type of receiver that is receiving the message.

For example, as we may be speaking right now, we are looking at a boa constrictor sleeping in its cage. It lives in a completely different world than we do, and we respond to similar stimuli in totally different ways. In fact, in some cases the snake appears to experience things that we have no or little awareness of and we are confident that we experience things that the boa has no personal experience of.

The same thing holds true in the practice of Tantra and what we are going to do here for a moment is demystify the entire word. Forget about its history for a moment, demystify it by simply saying that it is a method of self-transformation and a method of gaining more power over your self and the world you live in.

14

*If human beings are supposed to have hidden powers
why are they apparent in so few people?*

We have both discussed for many years Gurdjieff's *kundebuffer* concept which, in a very primitive sense, means "a lock."

It is a lock that prevents us—and possibly for our own "good"—from experiencing certain mental energies and powers and utilizing them.

This lock may have been given to us as a protective device until we, as a race, are ready to receive more information and cope with it, or it has been given to us as a lock to increase our, if you would, slave potential.

If you look at the history of the entire human race you can sum it up very simply as slavery. And what we mean by slavery is that man is a possession and is owned by various gods, by various governments and by various forces.

Most of all he is owned by the limitations of his own biophysical structure. Even the concept of the ego—which we are all deluded to believe means our executor, our executive, our personality—is "archetypal." That is, we all have one. Why?

If we are all deluded into believing that what we have is so unique and individual then psychics are nothing more than very good psychologists, because we all share most of our secrets in common. We all share the same issues, the same problems, and have many of the same skeletons in our closets.

15

If the obstacles are so great how can Tantra help get past them?

One of the purposes of Tantra is to help break down the formidable walls that have been constructed by ourselves, our biology, and our culture (which is the result of our biology interacting with various forms of environments whether they be so-called spiritual or so-called physical).

In terms of breaking down the walls that we have just referred to, the most important technique, as far as we are concerned, that's shared both by Hindu and Buddhist Tantra, is the idea of what we call 'de-programming.'

We use the word de-programming advisedly because we are not among those who believe a human organism is built in the image of a computer. But, considering the day and age in which this book is being written we think most readers will understand what we mean by this. (In the 1920's, serious studies of telepathy were referred to as "mental radio." In the early years of telephone, scientists used the telephone model to try to understand the operation of the nervous system.)

De-programming means *the removal of involuntary limitations*—the involuntary unrequested opinions you have taken as your own and have identified with the "true you."

These may be things like a political party or a Church or even the kind of food you eat.

Our own experience has been that, in terms of spiritual or psychological de-programming, *the most effective technique is the use of symbolism that represents evil or destruction in your culture.* To be sure, this does not necessarily imply criminal practice.

It *does* mean sacramental and magical practice with symbols; such as, in Western Magick, the inverted cross, the black goat or even the swastika. This last, of course, is a symbol of Eastern origin, with new Western meanings. If the reader finds these offensive, *that is exactly the point.* The fact that you use the swastika image *does not mean you embrace the philosophy of Nazism* or that you even embrace Satanism, although the philosophy of Satanism in the West has close correlations to Tantra in the East.

We pointed this out in a previous book: *Pacts with the Devil,* (New Falcon Publications, 1993, 1997) and weren't the first to do this.

A number of occultists in previous decades (for example, Dion Fortune) disliked Tantra because they considered it demonic Magick. They were quite correct (in a certain sense).

The idea is to work with these symbols to the point where they essentially don't mean anything to you anymore. In fact one is to create a forced nihilism in oneself, in terms of any meaning whatsoever, before rejoining the Universe as a meaningful structure.

However, this doesn't mean just staring at them or just meditating about them. It means actively invoking the power within yourself, calling up these spiritual forces, even performing black masses if you must. The important thing is the presence of a powerful emotional component, not just intellectual fixation.

In the sexual arena this can mean deliberately exploring practices and sex roles forbidden by your social milieu, or that you yourself find frightening.

For example, it is common among heterosexual men to fear being the passive partner in sex particularly if homosexual. This can be addressed by allowing your female partner to possess you (if you are a man) with a dildo.

16

What about secrecy in a country where religious freedom is the law?

By all means secrecy is essential.

America doesn't really have religious freedom. How many National Holidays do you know of that are not also Christian Holidays?

The goal of Tantra is to wipe away, through active battle, the chains, the bondage you were put into by your parents, the Church, the government and by the consensus trance of the culture at large. Since Tantra involves doing things that your neighbors might be shocked at, secrecy is important.

Letting too many people know what you are doing can get you into a lot of trouble. (For example, study the life of The Psychedelic Tantric, Dr. Timothy Leary).

If you go around wearing a T-shirt with an inverted Pentagram on it you could find yourself physically attacked by a fundamentalist walking down the street.

There is a great deal more person-to-person violence regarding religion than the news media reports and it is nearly impossible to get the police to respond to this sort of "hate crime" without absolute physical evidence.

However, what does come eventually from these practices is the realization that the group you are raised in is in a state of hypnosis, they are in a state of trance, a state of zombiehood. Historically, there is no more violent, anti-intellectualism and no more destructive religion in the world than Christianity.

Even Islam with all its attempts to conquer the world in the name of Allah has not been as destructive as Christian-

ity. The slave mentality of Christianity has held back
human progress by at least two millennia.

When you realize this and you see millions of people
going around saying how wonderful they are to each other,
constantly reinforcing the trance and then going out and
performing essentially criminal or cruel acts on other people, on their families and especially on their children, the
whole good/evil concept becomes meaningless. It becomes
a relative social issue.

It becomes that thing that fundamentalist Christians hate
the most: relative morality or situational ethics.

We were talking earlier about the void.

This is a good example of a low-level of realization of the
void: often that which you were taught was "good" becomes "toxic" and that which you were taught was "toxic"
is found to be "good." When you experience this, you begin
to realize just the sort of confusion you have been placed in
since you were a child.

This *sounds* like a simple thing to realize. And it is—in
your head. It is quite another thing to realize it in your gut,
in your deep psyche, so that it affects your behavior as you
deal with the world. It can be *very* shocking and unpleasant.

17

If the practice of Tantra changes one, how do the changes begin to manifest?

It has been our experience that under some circumstances using symbols such as the inverted cross, the black goat or the swastika, can cause strange and sometimes frightening events.

The active invocation of forces that can be considered demons or at least something that society as a whole does not want you to "socialize" with can lead to great revelation and release of energy.

You may have nightmares, fears, the running creeps, even paranormal events happening around you that are difficult to explain and appear completely irrational.

A number of people, including one of the authors, as a result of some of the practices described in this book have had machines break down around them (in one case, five brand new tape recorders within a 48-hour period). Some things just happen: cars stop, computers go down, keys disappear, old enemies appear, and you have a fight with your boss.

This is a low level of what might be called the "poltergeist phenomena." When you get to higher levels of this "phenomenon" and your silverware starts to fly around your room and your keys are missing *every* morning then— oh, well things have gotten out of hand!

Jokes aside, these are things you have to get used to.

Once you get past this point, if you have the nerve to do it—and *nerve and courage have to be cultivated*—you'll find yourself in a whole new world of feeling and thought and be able to deal with the average world more effectively.

On the downside, you may become increasingly alienated and disgusted with the people around you and find yourself having nothing in common with your friends and family.

In some Buddhists texts, the conversion to the Ultimate Buddha is often accompanied by a feeling of disgust (also know as the Gesture of Disgust).

In other instances you may find people becoming increasingly hostile toward you. This is another aspect of the work and will have to be dealt with in a sensible and productive way.

18

If I am looking for peace, why should I do something that produces fear?

A great Mage once said fear is failure and the forerunner of failure. In fact, if you do not feel fear you might have to question the effectiveness of what you are doing.

This is very important to keep in mind.

To feel anxiety and fear—as you are unlocking the key your mind, to forces that surround you and that are within you—have to create anxiety. It is a *must*. Must is a four-letter word and a very important four-letter word in this case. If your practice is working you will experience anxiety and fear. The first thing that people are trained to do, when they experience anxiety and fear, is to try to get rid of it. We suggest cultivating it and making it your dear friend.

This is why we have so many institutions today designed to get rid of anxiety and fear. And this is why we have so many failed institutions which have tried to control so-called alcoholism, drug addiction, and so forth. The attempt to remove anxiety and fear is natural in a production and consumption society.

When a society is concerned with production/consumption it cannot have its consumers occupied with their personal development; anxiety attacks, panic attacks, fear and trembling (to borrow from Kierkegaard). As such in your beginning practices you must accept fear.

Crowley's term "fear is failure and the forerunner of failure" simply means that one does not allow fear to prevent one from accomplishing one's ends. Fear is essential. Fear is a signal, anxiety is a signal, from the body and the brain to the *so-called you* that something is happening, something is working. Now, to run away from this is foolish.

To dwell on it is also foolish. To medicate yourself to death is also foolish.

Addiction is nothing more than hiding from the transmutation of the mind as it faces the void, as it faces the bridge.

19

Is all this stress necessary to this process?

A void is actually a bridge, sometimes a very shaky bridge.

It is very important to keep in mind that once you're involved crossing this bridge, from being *Homo normalis*—normal pathetic man—to being something more, to being higher, something better, you're going to run into difficulty.

You'll run into many difficulties. You may have difficulties with your job, difficulties with your children, your mate and so on.

Interestingly enough, these are some of the same warnings that Dr. Regardie used to give to patients who began their quest through neo-Reichian therapy or Orgone therapy.

He used to bring up that, as people progressed through the Reichian work or neo-Reichian work, they would often suffer indigestion, they would often suffer with impotency and they would often suffer from insomnia.

He used to call these "the three I's." He would warn his patients (and most of them didn't take him very seriously) that one of the results of breaking down the walls, (breaking the armor to use a Reichian phrase) is impotency, indigestion and insomnia—and loads of anxiety and fear.

20

What about the anxiety often reported accompanying Kundalini?

Having an anxiety reaction, which can hit unexpectedly, is sometimes an unwelcome effect of Kundalini.

Kundalini is a life-force that is not acknowledged to exist by most modern medical practitioners.

When Kundalini phenomena do occur in people spontaneously who aren't seeking it and do not have the education to know what it is (which is almost everyone) they're put on lithium, they're locked away, they're told they are having a psychotic breakdown, or told they are having a massive anxiety attack. All of this may be true from an orthodox medical or psychological point of view but it is not abnormal from the point of view of Kundalini.

To illuminate this answer further we will relate a story of a Kundalini experience that Mr. Black had recently...

A number of years ago because of circumstances in my life, I had a series of panic attacks. These are classically known as anxiety syndrome. They involved strong physical symptoms: the feeling of a band tightening around my solar plexus; an inability to breathe; numbing of the hands, the fingers and feet; rictus in my face.

I mention this only to demonstrate that I know the difference between an anxiety attack and something else.

Years later when I began investigating Yogic techniques in conjunction with Magick, which I had been practicing far longer, and began studying Tantra and Tantric techniques, I had several genuine Kundalini experiences.

One cold morning I was sitting at an Altar set-up in a state of deep trance. I had been adept at self-hypnotic induction for several years so there was nothing special about the situation. I found it very relaxing. It lowered my blood pressure and resulted in other good physical effects.

I was using as a meditation focus, aside from my usual rock crystal ball, a series of talismans that related to the elements.

Although I was physically cold, because of my state of mind it didn't matter. All of a sudden I became more rigid. My body—especially my torso—heated up. I felt flashing pains in my torso and portions of my hands and legs and I became covered with sweat. I first thought I was having a heart attack. I tried to move. I couldn't.

I felt completely paralyzed. This passed in about ten minutes. But the heat remained. That, too, passed eventually. I ended the meditation, checked my body and felt fine. I had had similar experiences with flashes like that before, with strange surges of energy, so I assumed this, too, would pass and the fear that I was going to die left me.

I had had a Kundalini experience and I discussed it with a friend of mine who practiced some of the same things I did and immediately identified it as a classic "tumo" experience.

(Tumo refers to the psychic heat that is is related to Kundalini and is produced by certain meditational practices that do not have any known "trigger" and occurs regardless of the temperature you are in or the activity of your body.)

I said thank you, fine. I didn't think anything of it because these things usually occur spontaneously and often there is no discernible result that lasts (which is often just as well).

I went to the gym to do my morning run which I normally did after performing the exercise I just described. As I was exercising I was so full of energy I felt like I was pumped full of methedrine. I ran faster and I ran longer and was absolutely filled with the most overpowering joy that I could possibly describe. By the time I was done I felt wonderful, I was emotionally elated and the elation stayed, I would say, for about a week.

The same sort of phenomena continued in terms of the energy and the feelings of joy and energies rushing throughout my body.

The following week I performed the meditation again and I made a change in the talismanic arrangement. This was apparently a mistake because I had another Kundalini experience but this time I felt like my torso was going to explode.

I literally felt my body had swelled to three times my normal size and generally speaking had a horrible emotional reaction to it filled with anger and despair and rage and when I ended the meditation I thought, 'well, this will just go away especially if I went to the gym and loosened up.'

I went to the gym to run as I normally did and felt awful. Absolutely horrible. My body continued to feel like it was going to explode. This is the only way I can describe the sensation. It wasn't a sensation of high blood pressure. It was a completely alien sensation to anything I had experienced before or since.

Mercifully.

This continued for several days. I was an emotional wreck; a physical wreck. Finally, I just put away all the talismans, anything that was related to what I was doing, and 'prayed' for the whole experience to go away.

Which eventually it did.

I personally have no doubt that what I had done was create a second arousal of the Kundalini force but this time in a way that energized portions of my psyche and portions of my body and probably portions of the so-called 'etheric' body—which is another thing that modern medicine does not acknowledge—that caused the phenomena.

21

If so many claim to desire psychic experience, why all the fear?

Because the fear is culturally induced. This literally means culturally designed and controlled.

This is where one has to be extremely careful and where one has to be willing to continue work after such an experience. Many people don't. We described in an earlier book *(Pacts with the Devil)* how we had seen many people who practiced magical and occult techniques and when, for the first time, get any supernatural results become absolutely panic-stricken and drop the whole thing.

They revert to "safe" practices like visualizing the 'white light' or Jesus. These practices are indeed safe—because they are inert. There are many people involved in magick and mysticism who, upon getting the 'supernatural' reaction they want, immediately run for cover. Some turn to everyday religion or take up fetishes and behaviors which are "rebellious" in form but harmless in essence.

This is unfortunate because they haven't been warned—either by books or by instructors—of what they have to deal with when these things happen. Fear of uncommon reactions is greater than we realize. Because of our culture, we are psychologically and physically unprepared to deal with such events and the side-effects of misfired Kundalini can be serious both medically and psychologically.

The downside to it is that you're not going to be able to find anyone to help you unless you're lucky enough to have a transpersonal psychologist as a friend or know an accomplished Yogi who can do something for you. One of the purposes of this book is to help correct this lack.

These emotional experiences are not only common for individuals who do magick, meditation and/or hypnosis. They also occur to people who are going through regular psychotherapy, particularly those going through one of the various forms of bio-energetic therapy.

We have disowned most psychotherapy because of its extreme social, political and cultural bias.

This has become particularly true in recent years when the housewives of America have decided that they have somehow gained the experience and powers to deal with the massive forces that reside in the collective unconscious and in the world at large.

Most individuals who have had psychic or Kundalini experiences are frequently thought of as being mad. And that might be true! However, to keep this in perspective, it is important to realize that the psychiatric/psychological community as a whole will diagnose most *any* person with such experiences as suffering from a psychosis or a personality disorder.

This is not something to be very concerned about unless your only form of assistance comes from the community at large. Keep in mind that Tantra is the inversion of what we Westerners consider community. This is why most Tantric practices take place in closed or sacred communities.

Most forms of in-depth work, whether Eastern or Western (other than the so-called "cosmic white light brotherhood"), is disruptive to all forms of community including many so-called Esoteric Orders.

Many individuals who evolve and change drastically while belonging to such an Order will find themselves thrown out or ostracized.

So you can just imagine what it would feel like for a person who belongs to what is regarded as an evil or an insane or crazy group to be experiencing things that even his *own colleagues* are horrified by.

22

How are such volatile practices held together in groups at all?

With a very great difficulty and usually due to the power of a Magical figure or Guru.

Tantric practice involves sex, power, physical practices and symbolic manipulations which are polytheistic in a monotheistic world and are culturally unacceptable, at least in a religious context.

You have to decide for yourself whether to work alone or to join a group.

23

How do you utilize a fragmented esoteric method?

We have seen the almost completely successful destruction of the Western esoteric tradition by Christianity and of the Tibetan traditions by the Communist Chinese. What there is left of it you can only find in the "grimoires" and legends of Black Magick that float through our history and the scant translations of the Tibetan material.

Most of these are ridiculously distorted. And, within the actual occult groups that do exist—even the ones with the very best intentions—they are always in danger of attracting people who have no social life, who want to consider themselves spiritually superior and fulfilled.

Many of these want comfort above all since we have all been trained to go to Church for comfort. For most people occult organizations are another form of Church.

A true magician is often a threat to any organization. These people either leave out of boredom and disgust or are shunted out by one excuse or another.

We have been witness to the sad deterioration of more than one movement, some of them quite large, into the most pathetic kind of little Church, and there is no talent left any more.

The people who run the organizations are mediocrities who don't want the personal emotional threat or stress of being surrounded by people with potential talent. As a result, it is to be assumed that until you make the acquaintance of someone or a small group of people who have the same goals you do you may in fact be more or less doomed to work alone for a while.

Most of the exercises in this book (and our other books) can be done either in a group or as an individual and theoretically, at least, most of the phenomena that occur can be dealt with in the same way. It is always good to have people to talk to without being afraid of some kind of unpleasant, petty little backlash.

Seeking out groups who are sincere and who are intelligent and run by people of genuine talent and genuine power is a good thing. We encourage this but always be aware that these groups are few and far between and many which started out exactly that way have unfortunately become something else entirely over time.

24

What about the idea of evil?

If you were to speak about "black Tantra" or the left-hand path of Tantra there is really a great confusion of terms from the Western perspective.

Tantra, while neutral from the perspective of those individuals who practice it in the East, is viewed as inherently evil and dark from the perspective of the Christian Judaic paradigm.

We must do a little qualification here. Many mystical Jews practice a form of "Tantra" or Sex Magick.

Certain Sufi groups also practice forms of "Tantra" or Sex Magick.

Even some secret Christian groups have a system of practicing Tantra or Sex Magick.

Getting back to the point, in our Western society whether you think you are practicing white Magick or black Magick, if you are practicing Magick *at all* it is evil from the social point of view. To repeat, becoming your own person and living your own life is the clearest definition of evil.

If you are practicing Tantra it is evil. There is no simpler way of saying it. Now, once we get within the groups themselves we are faced with a further division of the types of Magick and the types of Tantra that are practiced.

These are broken down primarily into our simplex, bipolar notions of good/evil, white/black, right-handed/left-handed.

We have observed some of the most intense arguments between practitioners of Magick and Tantra who have taken either the so-called black path or the so-called white path. These have been more intense and hostile than observed between born-again Christians and Magicians, or people who are "Wicca" or people who are pagan. This in itself is quite fascinating.

25

How does a person get past fear and trembling?

One of the authors (Black) has an acquaintance who spent more than 30 years in the Gurdjieff work. He was involved with a group in San Francisco and began this work back in the late 60's when Anton LaVey had started publicizing his Church of Satan (which has since become notorious or tedious depending on your point of view).

He became increasingly worried about the presence of so-called Satanic or Black Magick and this began to upset him. So his Gurdjieff teacher said, "Why are you worrying about this? Why don't you just go and see what they're about?"

He went to a lecture at LaVey's black house and when he came back he was rather confused and depressed. His teacher asked why. He said, "The only thing the man talked about was old carny tricks. He didn't talk about Magick or Satanism at all."

He seemed distressed by this possibly because he realized he had been deceived by his own fears and preconceptions.

To quote from a story of Mr. Black:

"Now, at the time I met this man I was re-reading some Crowley material. I forget which book it was but it had Crowley's sinister visage portrayed on the cover—and we started talking about 'black magic.' I said I had done things that were considered Black Magick and had gotten a great deal of personal profit out of them. And he said 'Doesn't it wear you out?' And I asked, 'What do you mean?'

He said, 'Black Magick.'

I said, 'What do you mean?'

He said, 'Black Magick.'

I said, 'How do you define Black Magick?'

And he said, 'Well, you know, Black Magick. Doesn't it wear you out? Doesn't it wear the practitioner out?'

That was the extent of the conversation. I could never get him to tell me what Black Magick meant.

I got the distinct image that practitioners were supposed to be worn-out scraggly looking husks rather like long-term heroin addicts as a result of these terrible practices even though he did not know what these practices were."

People are locked into concepts and fears which have to be broken down. The more you break your fears down the more enemies you will find you have, especially if you are foolish enough to talk about it as occasionally we have been.

The concept of black and white has very little meaning in Tantra.

The Tantric Buddhists of Tibet look with horror on some of the Bengali Tantrics of India saying they indulge in terrible vices, they use powers improperly, etc.

This is a result, in our opinion, that Tantric Buddhism in Tibet became public property—it became a public religion as well as a secret practice.

As a result, it had to concern itself, like any major religion, with regulating public behavior among the *hoi polloi* —the people with no particular talent, who lead their lives herding sheep or yaks or whatever the people in Tibet herd.

Even in Buddhism the concept of good and evil is irrelevant.

If a Tantric master is "good" it is because he feels like it. If he is "evil" he behaves accordingly because he considers that it is the way to behave under those circumstances.

However, he does not appeal to any outside judgment because Tantric Buddhism does not fear punishment by external gods. If you do not fear authority or do not admit that authority has the right to govern you, you are evil whatever your behavior may be.

26

Is it troublesome that Tantrism denies the authority of religion, yet deals with Magick, Supernatural Beings and Gods?

The real issue is simple. Authority for authority's sake—no.

The "worship" and the use of Gods—yes. It must be remembered that there is no single definition of what constitutes a God. Of course, the Christians would find this blasphemy.

The original Buddha himself is considered to have been an atheist. (This is not the same as a Western atheist who doesn't believe in anything.)

The Buddhists deal quite freely with ghosts and demons which they express as having the same kind of existence as any person. But, when you get into concepts of gods and universal punishment, the punishment is brought on by confusion and the inability to manipulate your mind and its relationship to the universe.

Among the Hindus, during the higher levels of initiation, the individual aspirant loses bit by bit the conditioning that was impressed upon him by parents and caste culture.

This, incidentally, is where the term "outcast" really came from—it came from being "out-of-caste," not from being "cast out." Someone who is out-caste is someone who no longer feels bound by the obligations he was told he had as a Brahmin, or a Warrior, or an Untouchable.

Knowing that these "obligations" were "arbitrary" or things he was simply saddled with, he begins to destroy them and then rebuilds himself.

This, of course, makes him extremely unpopular socially and this is actually what many initiates strive for. As a result, many of the higher initiates in Bengali Tantra—especially when they achieve greater and greater psychic, psychological and physical power—become figures of great fear to other people.

There have been a few circumstances where European ideas of evil were actually cultivated as a means of spiritual development in the East.

This was done especially with the "Thugs" who are famous in European legend and whose name has slipped into our language.

The "Thugs" were Kali worshipers who believed in propitiating the goddess by killing at random.

By doing so they believed that they were freeing themselves from the wheel of Karma.

People who think of Karma as a moral system are confused by this unusual belief.

In practice what the criminal sects were doing was becoming so bored, if you will, by acts of violence and crime that they freed themselves from the attachment to punishment. Today in the West they would be serial killers, psychopaths and high-ranking political figures.

If they felt no guilt they got no punishment. For them, Karma was a mental process that was largely brought on by themselves. Their cure for it, unlike the Buddhists, was to wreak as much destruction as possible until they were simply bored with the whole thing and no longer emotionally affected by it. At which point they stopped.

This is very similar to certain behavior modification techniques coupled with hypnosis, where the "undesired" behavior is practiced over and over again until the patient gets fed up with it and himself.

How much spiritual enlightenment this brought about we certainly have no idea and don't care to speculate.

The "Thugs" as far as we know have been dead for at least two hundred years, wiped out by the British Army.

This was a cult that existed for centuries and, some say, considered itself to be a valid Tantric sect.

The question of good and evil becomes very confusing and the question of Black Magick and White Magick also becomes confusing in the Hindu Tantras.

The same pattern doesn't apply to the Buddhist Tantras to the same degree.

In many Bengali texts there is a progression from the first section of the book to the last chapter going from religious devotion to the recitation of mantras. This can be looked at as either spells or hypnotic techniques depending on the mantra or your general attitude toward it.

At the end of the texts are presented rather violent magical practices which may be intended to harm a person perceived as an enemy or a hindrance.

This is especially true in the Kulanarva Tantra which is, among the Hindu Tantras, the one we have found easiest to read and understand.

At the beginning of the book you have Tantric and devotional practices to Shiva and Parvati. By the middle of the book they become more complex and deal with physical practices, dietetic practices and exercises to improve the Tantric adept.

At the end of the book what you have is a full blown "text of witchcraft" and instructions including those for making a doll of your enemy and burning it in a cremation ground with accompanying spells in order to destroy the enemy. Not so sweet and light as you've been told, is it?

So, clearly, from the Tantric point of view the more advanced adept is actually the more dangerous and wilder human being. This is completely alien to the American/European point of view which still (even unconsciously) uses the New Testament imago of Jesus as the model of the ideal person.

We mean of course, the mythical Jesus, who is an unemotional or mono-emotional individual who is incapable of reacting violently and is friendly to everyone and likes dogs and little children.

This is one of the most disturbing aspects of Tantra that has to be dealt with and that the individual will have to deal with within himself. He will have to, bit by bit; one by one, re-examine and re-judge everything he believes. You may find this far more difficult than you think. Because what we believe has little to do with what our life experience tells us.

27

What are some specific methods of deprogramming?

A movie, *The Mechanic,* which starred Charles Bronson and Jan-Michael Vincent, is an interesting example of moral neutrality and ethical precision.

Bronson, who was a hit man for the Mafia, was telling his young disciple Jan-Michael Vincent that "he lived in his head" and lived outside of common notions of morality and in this sense he was a master not only in various techniques and abilities but a master in the sense that he was in control of his own life.

At the end of the movie the disciple kills Charles Bronson leaving him with the idea that his primary mistake was his primary assumption, that he still needed permission to perform his acts of murder whereas Jan-Michael more or less stated, "I will do it when I choose, when I decide and when it's good for me."

Of course, in the end both were killed which reflects our moral movie mania. But the idea is clear.

One of the first exercises that we suggest for those who have not already done so is to purchase a Cross—a Christian Cross—and, using your own device and your own means, invert the Cross.

Put a chain or rope on it, put it around your neck and find yourself a relatively safe neighborhood like a downtown metropolitan area.

You are safer from the thieves than from most of your neighbors. So go downtown where there are thousands and thousands of people. Walk down the street and observe your own emotions and your own feelings as well as the reactions of others.

Particularly observe the emotions and feelings that you might believe are coming from others as well as their glances and stares at you.

This is a very important technique because it will place you out-of-caste or as an outsider. A person who must begin to learn to live in his own mind, if you would.

Another useful technique is to purchase a roll of quarters and, in a congested area drop a quarter every twenty seconds or so on the sidewalk; observe what happens.

If someone picks it up and offers it back to you refuse it saying, "That's not mine." Even if they claim they saw you drop it say, "No, that's not mine. That's not my quarter."

Continue to do it until all the quarters are gone.

Another very useful technique can be a bit dangerous and you will have to decide if you want to do it.

The danger here is not usually from other people but from hurting yourself by bumping into another person or some object. Preferably you should be alone. Shut off all music, television or whatever because they will assist you and we don't want you to be helped right now.

Right now we want you to do it yourself. After you wake up in the morning put on a blindfold. Take care of your morning duties and obligations, prepare breakfast for yourself, all with the blindfold on.

Live the entire day with the blindfold on. Do everything you have to do with the blindfold on. And then, later in the day, if you wish, turn on the TV. Listen to the TV. Listen to the radio, walk around.

Prepare and eat dinner. Get yourself ready to go to bed. Sleep with the blindfold on. In the morning when you wake up take the blindfold off and continue on with your normal day. Write down for later study everything you experienced the day and night before.

Another good technique for you to do at this time is make yourself a box lunch. Get a nice bottle. And if you're lucky enough find a fellow traveler and take them to your local cemetery; find yourself a very nice grave site and enjoy your lunch and have a very nice time in the afternoon; preferably a nice sunny day.

28

How do you deal with clashing realities?

The title of this section is "Meetings With Un-Remarkable Men." An interlude?

Sort of a satire on Gurdjieff's book.

In the beginning section of the book we told some stories about our own experiences, backgrounds, and theories of Tantra.

The principle question that needs to be answered, if you haven't answered it clearly in your own mind, is what are the benefits of Tantra and Tantric techniques and what it is that you are trying to change or escape by using them.

This may seem obvious to you yet some people are reluctant to admit to themselves the things that they really want to change, and are repulsed by how basic and common they are.

It is difficult to realize that many of these esoteric techniques are aimed at changing and controlling things that most of us consider to be rather ordinary and mundane. (Remember, that if there is a war in heaven it is between Stark Individualism and Collectivism.)

We will give you an example. Some years ago Mr. Black had an acquaintance who was a well-educated, friendly African-American man.

"I would see [him] socially when I lived in Hollywood. He wasn't really a friend but an acquaintance and we ran with the same group of people. As a result I saw him frequently. He was always friendly, with not a mean bone in his body.

Whenever I think of him, I am struck by one conversation we had a number of years ago. We were having cocktails after work in a bar and somehow (I don't remember the details of the conversation), I had brought up the fact that I didn't believe in Jesus or the Bible or something of that nature.

His first response was, 'Oh you are Jewish.'

I said, 'No I'm Irish.'

'Then you're an atheist.' He replied.

'No, I'm not,' said I.

And he stared at me absolutely at a loss to figure out what I was. Then he said, 'Oh, you're a Satanist.'

The truth was that at that time that was closer to reality, but not in the way he meant it, so I said, 'No, I'm not.' Well, this left him nowhere. He seemed absolutely confused. So I pulled out something (that was equally untrue) but it was closer to what he could understand, I thought, than any of the things I could say to describe my attitude.

I said, 'I'm a pagan.' (Well, that wasn't true either because at that time I had great disgust for the 'neo-pagan' movement.)

He just stared at me and said, 'What?'

I said, 'I believe in a multiplicity of gods.'

He said, 'You're a Hindu.'

I said, 'No.'

None of the labels fit.

For him, there were only three or four things that I could possibly be. I was either a Christian of some type, a Jew of some type, I was an atheist, or I was a Satanist.

When I said I was a 'pagan' it completely blew every circuit in his brain and he stared at me—his eyes literally bugged out—in absolute silence for almost three minutes.

I defused the situation by simply laughing and changing the conversation, so it may have been that he assumed that I was making a joke.

I was struck by the fact that this man's world was so constricted, his knowledge about the world around him so limited, particularly since this was Hollywood I was amazed."

Here's another example:
"Some years ago I was visiting my home in the Midwest and I did a Tarot reading for a friend of mine about a relationship he was having.

Well, I made it a rule then, as I do now, whenever doing things like that, never to have the person tell me the question I'm analyzing.

Why? Because, depending on how delicate it is, it can affect my willingness to stay with the cards or whatever forces I'm using. All of that aside I told him that the relationship would fail and this indeed came to pass in the time period that the cards described.

Instead of a straightforward reaction to this, his mother got wind of it, and from a simple demonstration of a divinatory technique that you could get from any psychic reader, I became a sinister sorcerer who cast a spell upon him and upon his girlfriend in order to destroy their relationship.

What they thought my motive for this was remains unclear. But the fact is these are people, who for the most part, would have flatly disbelieved any suggestion that I could do such a thing.

As soon as I demonstrated something as common as predicting the future (and premonitions and psychic predictions are among the most common psychic phenomena there are) then I was immediately transformed in their eyes into some monstrous demonic figure who could manipulate their lives without the least effort. I would be happy to believe that that were true; unfortunately experience tells me otherwise."

This kind of blind reaction, which often has absolutely no relationship to the circumstances involved, is the sort of thing that needs to be broken in yourself at the very beginning , and it is also a danger you must be on guard against from other people.

If you live in a fundamentalist community where you are completely happy and completely enclosed and never question anything around you, you won't even be reading this book. We hope.

29

Can you get addicted to Tantra?

Control your life in the direction you want to go, and free yourself of associations that are holding you back. If you are frustrated by a lack of ability to express yourself creatively, Tantra is an excellent way to proceed. But it can be dangerous, but rarely addictive. (The reason we say "rarely" and not "never" is that we know one person who gets addicted to *everything*. In fact, he's a high adept of a secret order.)

Another, more insidious kind of block, is the one that disguises itself as "healing" or "self-development." This is the *true* addiction—the one that kills.

In recent decades, twelve-step programs have been widely publicized and have generally received good press. Indeed, they may even help some people.

What is not widely known however, is the degree to which some of these programs, especially AA, regard their teachings as *literally* given by "God."

They will tell the person needing help that he can never be "cured," and must continue with the group for life, or he will *die*.

False information is given as medical fact in some of these groups, and many people are talked out of seeking desperately needed psychological help.

The people who enter these organizations are seeking freedom from one addiction. But they are not the heroes who beat the habit.

They find another addiction instead.

30

How can you avoid being normal?

This is the kind of thing the Tantric Adept must root out of himself. We all have things we want to believe and sometimes those things are negative and untrue and sometimes those things are positive and still untrue.

It is extremely difficult and may be impossible to form a complete balance, and certainly there is no such thing as complete objectivity.

But there's no reason to go through your whole life sunk in a complete trance absolutely divorced from actuality.

As fundamentalist Religionists ideate with their myths of worldwide Satanic conspiracies and their goal for world destruction... "He is coming to judge and make war," (19th Chapter of the Book of Revelations).

Or, as many business men do in their daily lives, going from cubicle to cubical in grade school, from cubicle to cubical in high school, to cubicle to cubical in college, to more little cubicles in the adult business world and then find peace and rest in the final cubical.

These men often deceive themselves believing that they know how the world works, yet it is the world which is working on them. They are helpless pawns who think that they are in charge.

Look at their apartments and suburban homes, all alike, doing the same thing, yet each thinking he or she is a unique self-driven individual.

People should only know what really controls them. If they did they would go mad.

31

*Is it bad to practice Tantra or Sex Magick without your
partner knowing?*

In this culture the choice is rarely there, particularly if
you are a man.

I (Dr. Hyatt) recall one time I was dating a young lady for
a number of months and we were having sex on a regular
basis. Unknown to her, I was holding certain mental images
and performing certain rituals in my mind while we were
having sex.

I never told her about this.

It caused her no harm or for that matter any good (we
think).

As time went on I began to think I might ask her if she
would like to be an active participant in these rituals.
Knowing all the potential problems that lay ahead I provided her with some books on various topics: religion,
psychology, philosophy and, of course, Tantra.

A few months went by and things were going fine
between us and I inevitably asked her if she would like to
be a participant in an experiment.

When she asked the nature of the experiment I explained
to her certain aspects of Tantra and Sex Magick and within
a few moments I noticed that a great silence had come into
the room and a very long face stared at me.

It was as if I had said something horrid or if someone had
just died. She looked at me intensely. She stared at me, she
opened her mouth but almost couldn't speak.

Finally she said, "You're talking about Black Magick
here aren't you?"

I said, "What?"

She said, "Black Magick. What you're doing is Satanic."

I said, "Well tell me what's Satanic about it."

She said, "Well, you're using sex for something it wasn't meant to be used for. You're trying to get power. You're trying to gain power. You're using me and my body to gain power so you can advance and get things you want in this world."

I said, "Well, what's wrong with that, particularly if you benefit as well."

She said, "No, I'm not that kind of person. I don't feel that way about it."

I dropped the conversation and we continued on our relationship having sex on a regular basis, doing things, going out together.

After a awhile I noticed there were more religious books (she was a Roman Catholic by origin) showing up in her home. Then after a while I noticed there was a Cross.

Then after another month I noticed there was a Cross in her bedroom. The message was getting through. She felt she was involved with a demon. And she needed the protection of the Church of her childhood upbringing to deal with the idea that she and I were going to take responsibility and intentionally perform a sexual magical act which would help us create power in ourselves and help us deal with some of our repressions.

So from an easy sexual relation with a Catholic girl I wound up in a situation where I was a demon and she was not just a girl raised as a Catholic—she was a practicing Catholic.

Sundays were no longer available for dates. We never went anywhere on Sunday. We never saw each other on Sunday. What was she doing?

She was going to Church.

32

How do names become spells and behavior patterns rituals?

Words are spells. Names are spells.

One of the principle techniques used in Tantra or, indeed, in any Magick, is the carefully constructed spell or mantra. When some European authorities were first investigating Hinduism and Tibetan Buddhism, they simply referred to mantras as "spells."

To a certain extent this is true. There are different types of mantras. And some of them have merely psychological effects and some of them, genuinely have paranormal effects.

Many scientists and sages maintain that the universe is living-vital information, in which case some words would be just as effective as machines.

In culture, words have been imbued with a certain type of psychological power. This is especially true of words which refer to things we identify with.

If someone says, "I am a Christian," that means that if you question the Bible or the historical Jesus you are directly attacking that person. It is personal.

Getting past this kind of thing in your own head is one of the most practical goals of Tantric techniques. Don't take your own beliefs personally.

We heard a story where a Black Magician told a Christian that Jesus was "nothing more than" a low-ranking Captain on an old space ship. You could imagine the reaction.

For example how would you like to be known, (1) as a toilet salesman or (2) the executive vice-president of sanitation? And here we see how names, just as in traditional witchcraft can empower, curse, or destroy. This methodology of name-"calling" is so common that it must go unnoticed.

We have known too many intellectuals who are fully aware of the "labeling" game but in reality refuse to allow this knowledge to penetrate into their daily lives, even for their own benefit.

But, remember, breaking the programming is only valid if you prevent yourself from falling back into it.

A technique Dr. Hyatt often used with people who were having severe anxiety reactions was to have them deliberately intensify the horrifying images in their mind.

He would tell them that if this intensification became unbearable to think of themselves and others wearing diapers.

Now, that sounds kind of funny or unusual or possibly even helpful. However, do you know something? Most people can not do it. Most people couldn't hold the image for more than a minute or two. What this means is that the power of will is easily sucked away by our day-to-day realities. (This is why sensory deprivation is an excellent way to get the brain accustomed to itself.)

Most people rarely used the technique in the real world. That is, when they were in a situation which required them to halt their conditioned emotional response (anxiety), they were incapable of employing the technique—or, for that matter, *any* technique.

This means that the loss of consensual reality *is* their anxiety. That is a very funny statement when you think about it.

Anxiety is reality for most people. Conditioned fear, conditioned anxiety. The normal day-to-day tension and anxiety is, in a perverse sense, desirable.

Go to a supermarket, go *anywhere,* people are tense. Like most animals in an open space, they get tense, they get nervous. The problem is not the tension or nervousness: the problem is that they do not recognize they are behaving like frightened animals.

Anxiety of this type is so common that we call it "noise." When there is a lot of noise the music recedes into the background and symphony of life can't be heard.

Now, getting back to the idea of imagining people in diapers.

The purpose of this image is to relativize you and the situation. It is to give you perspective and, thus, power. Many traditional and basic Tantric exercises of the mental type are just this simple. However, like mountain climbing, the execution is the hard part.

For example, you're talking to someone and you're very serious and very uptight and everything is on the line. If you're aware, you may feel all the muscles in your body tensing. Most people are so tense, nervous and neurotic that they don't even feel their own tension until the amount of tension is way beyond their average "baseline." It's like a full glass of water: one more drop makes it overflow.

Imagining a person in diapers activates your brain. It will put things into perspective.

There is another technique, developed many years ago by a great guru, who said, "Take your greatest worry, whatever it is, wherever you are, and hold your breath as long as you can. See what happens to your greatest worry, see what happens to your greatest fear, see what happens to your greatest anxiety."

You know something? People *can* do that. But how often do they apply the method?

This is why when you go into any bookstore you'll find thousands of self-help books on the shelves. They're all the *same book* and that is one reason why they sell so well.

Rarely does anyone apply the techniques or utilize the principles.

They've all been written a thousand times, a million times.
There's nothing new in them. What the books are really designed for is hope and time-consumption.
A person is feeling tension, they get a book.
They "read" it.
It takes up time.
A week or two after reading the book (unless in the mean time they've joined a Church or gotten something they wanted) they won't even know what the book had said; they escaped by identifying with the author and thinking of themselves as either a victim or someone more intelligent than most.

They don't apply the concepts. That is why authors get to write the same book over and over again and (some) make millions and millions of dollars. Few are capable of paying attention to the degree that is necessary to accomplish the task that is at hand and this is one of the profound things about *practicing real Magick or real Tantra or real Sex Magick*—or, for that matter, real *anything*.

The ability to focus and the ability to remember: Once you can focus and remember you can apply. If you cannot apply what you know it is useless except for an evening of dialogue, frustration and getting people excited by using words that offend them.

We do this as a technique; we do this quite frequently. We will just go into a social situation and we don't necessarily believe or disbelieve in anything the people are talking about.

What we will do is either pretend to believe completely and throw out a few key words that will make everyone like us and smile, or we'll take the words we know which will upset them and watch them get hysterical, nervous, tense, withdraw their smiles and turn their backs.

Thus the power of words.

The word itself is not the real issue. It is the identification of the person with the sound: thus the emphasis in Eastern discipline on silence and non-identification. Remember, everybody has an ego and the content of that ego is sound and noise.

So why bother taking the ego so personally, as if you invented it? The ego, in the sense of feeling personal, is extremely fragile. The ego itself is not fragile, but the feeling that it belongs to you—*is* you—is like fine crystal. This is why words, when identified with the ego, can cause intense emotional reactions, intensity to the point of murder—or a love affair.

33

I have read a number of your books and I find them stirring but I think you are prejudiced. How do you see yourselves in this matter?

Prejudice is just a buzz word for arrogance.

Playing with words can be a great "blessing" or a great "curse." You can communicate with them, you can have fun with them. However, you can also kill with them—or you can be killed.

When we talk about people being confused by titles and being unable to visualize their parents in their underwear it makes things seem rather silly and/or at least not earth-shaking. In fact, this is a major human problem. And it is, in fact, the principle danger any aspiring adept has to deal with and has to face, while at the same time breaking out of his own shell of programming.

He has to be very wary of his own environment and his own personal safety in terms of who knows about what he is doing. In this sense, we are all secret agents. Fleming was a Tantric master.

This is one of the reasons for secrecy in the practice of Magick or in the practice of any of the esoteric arts. There are other compelling reasons as well.

For example, one of the nastiest syndromes in any society under stress, especially one with competing classes (and we don't mean this in the Marxist sense, although economics always has a great deal to do with this) is what we call the "at least I'm not" syndrome—at least I'm not a nigger, at least I'm not a faggot, at least I'm not a kike—or put it in the reverse: at least I'm "saved," at least I've got a job, at least I've got a wife and family.

What this has to do with dealing with people and breaking down programming is a simple question we ask ourselves when dealing with extreme types of people who are locked into what we would consider a ridiculous maze of mental concepts like religious fundamentalism, and we stop and ask ourselves, "What else have they got?"

At the base of all identification is non-identification, a feeling of free float—which is the essence or base of all personality. After all, personality is outward appearance and people see themselves as they imagine others see them. Behind personality lies great powers which some call "natural" until they get out of hand and upset your neighbor. For example, lust, greed and sex are the engines which sew the costumes called personality.

How many people do you know who have conquered these forces, that is put them to use in their own service?

The question here is who is the man behind the screen? The answer is simply force itself twisted by events and causes to manifest itself in a particular form. That is: Who you are. That is the purpose of any true system of development. Even the self-help books rely on these forces, the how-to books are, in fact, simply getting this or getting that—money, power, sex, the sale, the new body, etc. This is the truth of mankind—he is a show off in denial.

34

Does Tantra have a view of the Universe?

Yes, many.

Broadly speaking, the Tantric view of time and history is cyclic rather than linear. It utilizes as tools such things as astrology, human and animal sexual cycles as well as many other methods to judge appropriate action.

It will be noted that the above-mentioned tools are divinatory; that is, they are dynamic rather than static.

But more than divinatory, the cyclic and dynamic point of view affects how a person sees himself and what he does with himself. Not only is time different but as such so is space. While these ideas seem abstract they, as much as gravity, affect all of human behavior.

The Jesuits were excellent at using time and space models coupled with dogmatic reason and logic to twist you about in order to force you to accept their primary principles and values, most of which were patently absurd.

It is very important, then, that while you learn to take things seriously, at least in terms of your own experiments, that you have a good sense of humor particularly when you find yourself constructing a cosmology—a world view that is a result of your experiments and experiences.

It's hard to become a true-believer if you don't believe truly. And this is one of the major issues of society (which is nothing more than groups of individuals): that each person has to act as if his beliefs and actions are, indeed, True with a capital "T".

Only Adepts are capable of putting on truth as a woman puts on shoes. Once the "truth" is worn out they toss it.

The constructs of identity and personality are illusions in the normal sense of the term. They are, in fact, created from one's wants, needs and desires much as one would create a building. And tension is like the mortar which holds the bricks of the building together.

The thing Dr. Hyatt used to say to people who drank too much is the guy who got drunk in the evening is not the guy who had the hangover in the morning.

If you drink a lot you're going to have a hangover and there's no battle with alcohol in this case. Alcohol is a chemical and it is indifferent to you—it doesn't care about you. You care about *it*.

Identity is based on multiple matrices of opposition. Give people what they claim they want and they will die—conflict ceases.

35

Is the focus of Tantra spiritual or physical?

Tantra is physical *and* spiritual. Easy answer?

It involves health and physical practices as well as mental disciplines.

There is, in Tantric theory, no division between the physical and the mental. People who have taken the trouble to practice bear this out.

Many of them who make the discovery the division between mind and matter is artificial don't like what they feel, see or experience. They are holding on to their old habits. Usually they will drop the practice.

There is nothing more common than intellectualist spirituality.

This is partially a holdover from Christianity (which represses almost all activities except those in service to the Church) and also from Victorian scientific reductionism.

Most people don't realize that, in spite of the fact they have had an education and "think" they live in an enlightened scientific age, *if they are lucky,* they are really living in a sixteenth century model of the universe.

And, in terms of basic material views, they are no further ahead than the middle of the nineteenth century. In other words, what people think they understand in terms of the laws of physics...they don't.

Most people involved in esoteric practices have a tendency to be very un-physical and very unhealthy. The principle example that always comes to mind is that of the so-called "neo-pagan" community.

We do not consider ourselves neo-pagans because we are not particularly interested in gods or goddesses except as *devices.*

However, what strikes us is the contradiction—the obviously, painfully, embarrassing contradiction—between the behavior of people and what they claim to believe.

For example, if you are familiar with Wicca and other neo-pagan groups who claim to be perpetuating the so-called "old religion," you may be aware that many practitioners have severe problems with clinical obesity, physical cleanliness, chain smoking, bad eating habits, and a host of other things; and all of this in people who claim to be nature worshipers and in tune with nature.

There's also a massive amount of ego inflation, backbiting, infighting and dogma used essentially to get people who have no life outside the group into high power positions in the group. For most of these people we would suggest one thing: lock away all the books they've got on Wicca and get a gym membership.

This may seem crude and unspiritual but we have found from personal experience that this is the best thing you can possibly do.

Physical exercise, especially aerobic exercise, has startling effects on thinking as well as feelings.

Once you learn to go into trance or trance-like states *while exercising* you might find some remarkable things happening emotionally as well.

Tantra in both the Hindu sense and the Buddhist sense involve the cultivation of the body.

In Hindu Tantra it has to do with Hatha Yoga. Hatha Yoga is a very complex system, and takes more than "two weeks" to enlightenment and a new body.

We recommend that exercise and meditation be done as often as possible. As Robert Anton Wilson says, "Do it every day."

36

Are the meditation techniques as complex as some Eastern sources imply?

The problem with primary sources from the Orient is two-fold: cultural misunderstanding and not knowing the underlying basis for the material. In other words, are we in the 1st grade or in graduate school? This translates into what book do you chose to match your knowledge and ability?

We have learned that people involved in the Occult, when faced with the specter of hard work, will probably stop in their tracks. The English translations of the Oriental texts make the task seem even worse than it is.

If you can get past this barrier it will be of enormous service to your development, your view of yourself and your way of dealing with the environment and the people around you.

My own (Jason Black) experience with it came as a result of doing extended work with trance induction states. I started out using techniques of hypnosis and when I no longer needed the hypnotic induction techniques it developed into straightforward meditation.

A lot of people will object that hypnosis and meditation are not the same but, as Alan Watts pointed out, most mediation states are hypnotic states and a great deal of trance induction through Yoga, through mantras, through drumming are considered to be traditional hypnotic inductions.

The principle difference between traditional hypnosis and the mediation state is that in hypnosis you have *guidance* (e.g., by the hypnotist, a pre-recorded tape or yourself).

In the mediation state the trance is left alone to float. These trances can be of varying depths from one where you're very relaxed and immobile (which is the most common one), to one where you go into an almost somnambulistic sleep in which you have no conscious thoughts or dreams and wake up anywhere from a second to an hour later feeling completely refreshed, often with spontaneous healing within your body and a totally different emotional and intellectual flow.

This kind of practice eventually led me (Black) into using exercise as an adjunct to meditation. I usually meditate for an hour and then go to the gym. I have been able to maintain trance states well enough and thoroughly enough that, while running, I essentially was in a trance—lost all sense of time, lost all sense of effort—and increased my running distance and strength far more quickly than I should have under most circumstances. I did this without pain, without stress and without injury.

37

Why don't we experience that mind and body are one?

We do.

It appears that we don't because of religio-cultural training and a placebo effect (post-hypnotic suggestion). With tongue in cheek we are saying, "because the Bible told you so!" (Or as Lewis Carroll put it, "What I tell you three times is true.")

The simple notion of mind and matter is really a question of measurement. Now think about that. Basically what we call matter is something we can measure. Basically what we call mind is something we cannot measure *as well.* O.K?

So consider that in light of the experiments of some Hindu physicians who have come to the West and are trying to create a sort of scientific Yoga cult by using EEG measurement and the like to "prove" to the so-called Western pseudo-intellect that what they're dealing with is not simply pure suggestion.

For some strange reason people find the idea of suggestion degrading to their pride, intellect and sense of self. Why? Americans in particular think of themselves as self-starters, great thinkers and masters of the keys to the temple.

38

How does one use Imagery as a device?

Let's talk about sex.

One of the most important elements in bio-physical and physical self-development is masturbation.

Masturbation?

Something in which we believe and which we hope all of you have done.

Masturbation can be used in a very profound fashion. And this is what we call the "death-of-self." That's a real fancy title!

The technique of masturbation to achieve the death-of-self is simply this: first develop a beautiful image of yourself. If you're heterosexual and are attracted to the opposite sex, convert the image to one of the opposite sex. Otherwise, leave the image alone.

Then masturbate to that image.

For example, suppose you want to lose weight. If you're a heterosexual male, imagine yourself as a beautiful female. Imagine that's it's actually you but with feminine characteristics; while this is often difficult and may be a bit advanced at this stage in your development, begin to masturbate to this image of yourself as the opposite sex not in the physical form that you're in but in the physical form you would like to be. Make the image so beautiful that you want to make love to it.

Let's suppose you're thirty-five pounds overweight. What you need to do is to develop a female image of yourself that is ten pounds under your weight or twenty pounds under your weight or thirty pounds under your weight or a hundred pounds under your weight—whatever works out for you.

Then begin to masturbate to that image you've created. (This may be difficult at first because most masturbation is involved with fantasies having to do with simple sexual frustration.)

In summary: if you are a male who is thirty pounds overweight; pretend you're a female thirty pounds overweight. Then, make yourself beautiful, give yourself a beautiful face, give yourself a beautiful body and then concentrate on that image and masturbate to orgasm.

This could take you six months, it could take you a week, it could take you a year or maybe you will never to be able to do such a thing. These are some of the techniques that you can do in your mind that violate the programming process of our entire society.

If you were to read a thousand books you would probably never find this technique mentioned. It is very ancient and potentially dangerous. The reason I say this is that a lot of people have unfounded fears of homosexuality. But just because you have homosexual fantasies or homosexual desires does not mean you are going to become a homosexual. Or vice versa.

Our society has caused us to take our androgynous self and turn it into a personality, an identity, something we can hold onto.

Why do you think people beat up homosexuals? Do they hate them? We don't think so—they don't even know them. They beat them up because their very existence is a threat to their false notion of personality, to illusion.

Think about that; re-read what you've just read. Think about it very carefully. This is one of the most powerful techniques you will probably find anywhere. And the most difficult.

You may now understand that we call it the masturbation technique of death-of-self because it is a very great ego death for a person first to visualize themselves as a member of the opposite sex, and second to make love to "it."

Another mental imagery technique that is used in traditional Hindu and Buddhist Tantrism (and to a certain degree in traditional Hermeticism), involves the use of a vivid or intense mental image. (For some people it may be easier to use a photographic image or a graphic image.)

For example, find a selection of photographs or drawings depicting people whose health and beauty you want to imitate. (It is important that the pictures not be of people you know personally.) And, while there should also be an erotic element to the image, that isn't primarily the point.

The primary point is to meditate on something that radiates health and beauty. During the course of your meditation you should instruct yourself using standard hypnotic techniques to absorb all the information—both physical and mental—that these images convey to you. In time your body and your mind will come to imitate them.

This is a more orthodox variation of a Tantric technique where the image is seen and mentally drawn into the body. In other words, the image of the god or the pin-up or whatever you want to imitate is literally drawn into the body and absorbed so deeply that the qualities of the image are brought into your system.

This technique can also be used to eliminate undesired behaviors and qualities. This works remarkably well and in surprising ways.

Keep in mind that these techniques emphasize the doing not intellectual understanding because, as with any machine, understanding of function is not required for operation.

39

Is backsliding a natural process?

In a book by Dr. Charles Tart (a professor of psychology as the University of California at Davis) is a discussion of the Gurdjieff work called "Waking Up".

Tart said that the first time he tried one of Gurdjieff's waking up exercises he was profoundly impressed by the results he got—and then he forgot to do it again for three months.

This is very typical. You forget to do "it." Your "super-ego", to use a Freudian term, doesn't want you to do "it." You're a bad little boy if you do it. So things happen. You forget, you get sick, you oversleep, you twist your ankle. You decide that your work schedule is so heavy that it interferes with your physical work at the gym or with your meditation. Etc.

You feel that you simply have to drop it for a time and you simply end up dropping it forever.

This is our defense mechanism at work and, like most defense mechanisms, it does not appear to us consciously. You have to understand that we are not one "self," we are many.

In Gurdjieffian terms the work of the adept is to *create* a self. In Buddhist terms it is to eliminate the false selves and unite more and more and to absorb more and more of the world at large within yourself. This is the explanation for the miraculous feats of the Buddhist monks who have absorbed more of the universe within themselves. They are more a part of the whole universe than the average person who is locked into illusion.

In Indian Hindu Tantra the goal is "energy." The Kundalini has to rise through the system and to accomplish this you must eliminate all the blockages that shunt the Kundalini off in the wrong directions—directions that make you neurotic, that make you depressive.

This is one of the reasons some gurus make you change your name and wear a robe of the same color as that of his other students.

To Western eyes this deliberate conformity is the worst kind of behavior. Of course, there is no more virulent cult of conformity than Christianity. But that is completely ignored. It's the surface things that are looked at.

40

If you say there is no distinction between mind and matter what of the doctrine of the soul?

First of all neither science nor philosophy can answer the question of what matter is. Thus, in one sense, it is ridiculous to even speak of a soul.

Gurdjieff even went so far to say that people do not have souls, but can develop them through effort.

The doctrine of the soul in Christianity is one of the great deceptions and the great tools for manipulation.

You have one soul and one lifetime.

You're going to go to hell or heaven.

You've got to do exactly what we say and you have to do it now.

Ironically, for the Buddhist Tantric and to a great extent for the Hindu Tantric (although the Hindus believe in the "Atman" and the Buddhists do not) you have no self, yet you have many lifetimes. This sounds very confusing but to the Tibetan Buddhist there is such a thing as a "knower."

41

What of my personality? What is it?

The personality is "evil" because it is a cluster of "accidents."

In fact the personality is a waste of time, except insofar as it serves the purpose of the Adept.

How many of us have personalities that fully serve our purpose? Very few, although some of us are lucky enough to have personalities that serve our purpose some of the time. For them the "knower" continues and is reincarnated in another body.

If the Adept has worked properly and has absorbed enough of the universe—enough of the dharma—and has done enough of the work, it becomes a greater being—a greater "knower"—so that in the next incarnation it is more brilliant as a human being. Artificial influences forced on it by other people are more easily sloughed off.

In "playing" with your personality, you may find it useful to employ images of others as mediation devices. You can use these images to change yourself. The chances are that those images are so different from the "you" that your family or friends are familiar with that you may be ridiculed if they knew in what way you were using them.

Institutionalization has happened in some circumstances (believe it or not; you wouldn't believe what some people are legally put away for if somebody really wants to do it.) The images themselves can certainly be kept in the open if you want to, but the religious and devotional use must be kept secret except among people who are your colleagues and share the same ideals and goals.

You may learn (as many people have found), that in trying to improve yourself, you will create enemies. Often, the worst enemies are your families and friends because they may become extremely uncomfortable and the world may seem out of control for them to see you change. Nowadays, in pop-psychology terms, this is called "co-dependency," and in rare cases, "symbiotic psychosis."

In any family system (and you can look at families as the many cells in *you,* or as the actual people in your real family, or as your friends), you have what is called the "identified patient." The identified patient is also known as the "trouble maker."

The identified patient carries the pathology of the entire family to the point that they can't stand it so they send him to therapy.

The therapist gets him better but the rest all get sick. And so they do everything in their power to make sure the identified patient remains crazy.

To be more specific and down-to-earth the "patient" then becomes the identified victim. As long as the victim or patient remains the object of the pathology of the system, all the units of the system remain intact and "functional."

Each piece balances the other. If you begin to change and *show* that change, the entire system begins to collapse. This causes anxiety because your personality is an anchor for everyone else's personality and vice versa.

If your personality changes, their personality is deeply affected. This affect occurs because personality and individuality is, in itself, very tenuous and inter-dependent. So, in psychotherapy, when the so-called identified patient or "the sick one" starts to become better, everybody joins in to help them *remain sick*—and possibly get sicker.

One common factor among all great developmental systems is to be very careful about who you hang around with, and who you base your identity on. This "simple" social fact is the principal basis for the rise of monastic systems in various traditions. These include the initiatory schools of the Egyptians and Greeks. (In the beginning, these "schools" were physical buildings where the initiate could live apart from others who lacked his talents or commitment.)

If you are among a group of people whose identity is a partial function of *your* identity and your changes affect them, they may try to destroy you in unconscious ways.

This is not personal, this not paranoia, so don't get lost by taking it personally or becoming paranoid yourself. This is a mechanical process no different than the orbiting of the planets around our Sun. If one changes the others are affected.

So a very important thing in Tantra is to learn how to maintain illusions: learning how to become a good actor or a good actress, learning how to walk on the stage, learning how to walk off the stage, learning how to take bows, learning how to receive applause, learning how to give applause.

These concepts are very offensive to normal people because normal people do not want to believe that anybody is acting or putting something "on", especially them. This is how tenuous and threatened their personality really is. They really need to believe in the illusion of who you are in order for them to believe in the illusion of who they are.

The Buddha was very clear on this and we always remember when he said "Why ask where the arrow came from that is in your chest? Why ask who made it? Why ask who shot it? The first thing you do is to fix it, to remove it, to heal it."

This form of ultimate spiritual pragmatism flies in the face of almost every religion and the various definitions of matter and spirit; individuality and collectivity.

Jung developed the idea of the collective unconscious which sort of implies that we all have images of this or we all have images of that and we all even have a collective image of self.

That is stunning when you think about it. That collectively we all have an image of individuation, or individuality as part of the collective unconscious which, in turn, includes the so-called ego that you are identified with and that you act out with.

Really, you see, you are an actor but you don't know it. Your personality, your way of behaving—you have been made an actor without being a director and without being a producer. And this is very important to keep in mind. You need now to become an actor as well as being the director and the producer.

42

Can verbal affirmations be as useful as images?

A positive mental attitude is pragmatic under most circumstances unless it represses anger and feelings of oppression. However, and this is most important, an attitude of any kind is like a sheath. It is superficial, and as such can not stand the test of extremes.

When a person is, say, optimistic or pessimistic, you must first ask the question of *why they need to have an attitude at all.* This will reveal what underlies all affirmations including those used by the Christian Scientists and the "I Am" cult.

So-called affirmations can be useful but those of us who know people who have spent their lives in Christian Science or in Science of Mind know that thinking happy thoughts doesn't always cut it.

The use of images is holistic—it covers beauty, it covers sexual attraction, etc.—and, if the image is properly selected (i.e., it has deep meaning for you), and has emotional impact on you, it will also have intellectual impact. The reverse, however, is rarely true.

The effect of the technique of masturbating to a perfected image of yourself is much more powerful than any happy thought or positive mental attitude.

Orgasm covers your body, your mind. It temporarily paralyzes the nervous system—the French call it "the little death"—and completely absorbs your attention. Now, orgasm isn't always necessary for the absorption of an image of this sort, but infatuation is. By infatuation we mean fascination on many levels—almost love.

Many Tantric practitioners have love relationships with these images that are sexual in nature. One of the authors had a trance experience where "astral sex" took place with a "spirit" called up from an old book. The effects were such that, while sitting perfectly rigid in a trance, he experienced bodily reactions as though he were being touched by another person.

In Western Magick this is called involvement with an Incubus or Succubus and many magicians consider it a form of psychic vampirism.

This kind of experience can be very startling and is indicative of a degree of closeness to an image or being that indicates real progress. On the negative side it can also lead into obsession (in the religious or occult sense).

43

Purity is often mentioned in Yoga and religious disciplines. Is it important in Tantric practice?

Regarding the subject of purification, which often comes up in any kind of Yoga, self-development, and even the occult, our own experience has been that ritual purification habitually done over a long period of time, has a profound psychological effect and is a very important part of any committed activity.

It is very useful to do certain exercises each day for the purpose of psychic and physical purification.

These are very effective in dealing with environmental influences, because the more psychically and physically sensitive you become, the more you increase your personal power in manipulating the world and improve your invulnerability under certain circumstances of stress.

Most of the European "grimoires" contain instructions for what is called "the bath of the art."

Usually, these instructions are completely ignored. For our part we find that using one of these short simple rituals before bathing in the morning is a very effective way to cleanse your mind and may also have a real psychic effect.

For our part we have used a ritual from the Constitution of Honorius (see *Pacts with the Devil.* 1997). Most of the existing manuscripts are in French and like most "grimoires" it's a combination of what the authors call "from elsewhere": folk Magick, Cabalistic ritual and a few gleanings from Cornelius Agrippa.

In any case, whether you take a shower or take a bath the ritual cleansing for the morning is done in this manner: run the water, either filling the tub or turning on the shower and stand before it without getting in.

Imagine white light infusing the water and the room, reciting this prayer or some variation of it if you don't like the various God names or religious orientation;

"Lord God Adonai who has created man from earth to reflect thine own image and likeness, who has created me also unworthy as I am. I pray thee [here you make a equilateral cross—not a Christian cross—using your hand or a wand or whatever tool you like] to bless this water that it may be healthful to my body and soul that all delusion and ill will may depart from me. O Lord God, almighty and ineffable who didst lead thy people forth from the land of Egypt and didst cause them to pass dry shod over the red sea, grant that I may be cleansed by this water from all my impieties and may appear blameless before thee. Amen."

Enter the tub or the shower and cleanse yourself, and at some point if you're in a bathtub full of water hold your nose and immerse yourself completely head and face under water, rise out of it and say "asperge me with hyssop O Adonai, and make me white as snow."

This is a variation from the Song of Solomon. If you are in a shower you do essentially the same thing after you have cleansed yourself. Step out of the shower and imagine your body suffused with a cleansing white light.

As an alternative to both these methods, after you thoroughly cleanse yourself, go into your bed room or living room and face East and imagine a ball of white light in front of you. Then turn to your right (South), and imagine a ball of red light. Turn again to the right (West), and imagine a ball of blue light. Turn again to the right (North), and imagine a glowing ball of saffron light. Finally, turn to the right again (back to the East), to close the circle.

Imagine these long enough to solidify them and imagine them hovering about you for the rest of the day. Then forget about the matter.

At this point our own practice involves a period of divination. This is not only a good habit to cleanse your mind and prepare yourself for the day but it is an excellent way to test increasing psychic abilities that may develop from these practices.

Jason uses Tarot cards as he's used them since he was 15 years old. However, you may use any fairly complex system of divination you like.

The I Ching is an excellent example and requires very little in the way of preliminary learning.

The Tarot, on the other hand requires a great deal of practice and a great deal of memorization, although a book can be used for beginners.

If you choose to use the I Ching all you really need is three coins. (If you're a purist you can use I Ching coins.) We use three dice marked with either three dots or two dots on each side. The I Ching is perennially in print (any good edition will work well), and can be purchased in most good book stores.

Divination is something the practitioner ought to do every day unless prevented by some unavoidable obstacle It takes very little time and it allows you to start your morning with a clear head. This is over and above any serious meditation practices that are more time consuming;

As an adjunct to the purification there's the question of diet. A great many Yogis and Easterners as well as Western ceremonial magicians have adopted vegetarianism out of philosophical principles. For our part we don't think the wily hamster of the forest is our brother. So we find the philosophical notions trivial. We've also observed that most of these people, while they do maintain a strict vegetarian or lacto-vegetarian diet, are not always healthy.

For example, you can eat a large bag of potato chips every day and maintain that you are technically a vegetarian while packing your arteries with enough fat to kill you by age 55.

There are also problems with lactose vegetarianism. Many compensate for the lack of meat by eating lots of cheese and eggs. The fat content of these can be killing on the body.

For our part, while we always try to watch our diet to a certain extent, we never had an aversion to meat or became vegetarians. However we found that after six months to a year of doing deep trance work, (that is, auto-hypnotic meditation and doing the techniques of purification and divination), we discovered that we had a lack of desire for meat for a time.

All of this happened quite automatically. Now, anyone who gets involved in this needs to make some effort concerning their diet because many people we know in the occult field, especially Western occultism, are in terrible health.

A lot of this will strike the typical participant in the occult as unpleasant and as something they are unwilling to do. But we can't emphasize strongly enough the importance of bodily involvement in doing this work. *This is not exclusively mental work.* Everything you do has to be physically involved. There is no bifurcation, there's no dividing line between the spiritual and the physical.

This is what the Tantrics and magicians teach more than anything else. Our own experience with ceremonial Magick and psychism in general is that spells—which seem so ridiculous to the modern mind and are seen as largely symbolic—if done as closely as possible to the original instructions, work. And they work better than any simple mental visualization or exercise possibly could.

44

What are the "psychic accidents" people talk about?

Some of the so-called disasters we've experienced have been of a spontaneous nature and seem to have involved either a technical mistake on our part or quite simply an unforeseen circumstance with the invisible forces or principles that we were working with. Remember, these forces have their own set of rules.

One technique for dealing with undesirable emotional or psychic phenomena is, in Tibetan Buddhist terms, "vanquishing." This method involves direct opposition.

Vanquishing, more or less, is self-explanatory. You identify the difficulty. You identify the undesirable behavior. Depression, for example, is certainly a sign that something is wrong.

In the vanquishing technique, you form a meditative exercise or spell (in the classic Western occult sense) that sets up a force opposing the principle you want to be rid of.

If you're going to use this kind of technique, be prepared to spend a very long time at it and commit yourself to doing it on an almost daily basis. You'll find that remarkable results occur, but you will also find that you will have what we call collapses or crashes: you will have a long period of success and then, whatever the principle or behavior you are working on may have been, tends to re-assert itself in full force. This has to be taken calmly, without attacking yourself and *without guilt.* You simply begin again and you will find that eventually the exercise will work.

45

Many religious and Yogic techniques say to suppress
anger and hate? Is this true of Tantra?

Hate!

One thing one usually wants to avoid socially is using the four letter word "hate."

These days we all prefer to use the other four letter word called "love."

The history of mankind really doesn't embrace either of those notions except as political and psychological tools to manipulate the middle and lower classes. And politically, of course, is when we have an enemy who is out to destroy the good (another four letter word) and the good is always "you and me" and the evil (another four letter word) is always somebody else.

The power of hate is overwhelming. In fact it is so overwhelming that there are few magical, religious, or philosophical traditions that embrace the power of hate and learn how to manipulate it.

To hate with one's entire being is one of the greatest virtues, as it forces you to look at and face some of your deepest desires.

To leave no deed unpunished means to do harm to anyone who harms you. It has the same effect as "love thy neighbor" as yourself, except it helps you face the most unacceptable truth, "hate yourself as you hate your neighbor." This, of course, is a technique, *not* a moral principle, and should be dropped as soon as you've gotten over your revulsion to the idea.

The whole idea of Tantra is to turn things upside down. This is a fundamental step.

46

Can you explain the concept of Inversion?

You will see kids on the streets with green hair, wearing shorts on their chests and t-shirts on their lower torsos and mixed shoes driving motorcycles with all sorts of strange colors on them.

There is nothing wrong with this inversion except that it's out of control. And it's purely reactive. This is one of the keys. Purely reactive emotion and hatred inevitably leads nowhere but back to its reactive origin.

As it is often said, the hippies of the 1960s are working on Wall Street, buying bigger and bigger houses, trying to embrace the middle-class values they attempted to reject during their bio-chemical reactive phase.

Tantra will destroy your notion of purity.

It will also destroy your notion of your worthlessness because both are nothing more than vanity.

In essence ideas such as these form a corpus of vanity without the will or the tools to make your dreams come true. Making dreams come true requires power.

47

Some Gurus have been criticized for the accumulation
of wealth and power, while Christian Priests claim
poverty. What is the Tantric position on the
accumulation of worldly power?

Poverty is one of the great powers for, through it, the
Priests suck you dry.

Power is not sinful to the Bengali Tantric system.

One purpose of this book is to blend the Bengali and the
Buddhist together and also to blend it with Western occultism.

Western Magick had the same components that Eastern
Tantrism has always had in terms of its intellectual depth
but much of that was destroyed by Christianity.

Power is not a part of Buddhism for a sound historical
reason. If you read the Buddhist Tibetan books the goal is
knowledge and, of course, the Buddhists are pacifists.

Our opinion is that this is an historical luxury. When
Padmasambhava brought Tantric Buddhism to Tibet in the
seventh century it was a barbaric violent nation. Now, since
the communists have invaded it in this century, it is worse.

Because the Buddhist Tantrics were protected they had
the luxury of being pacifists.

They had the luxury of claiming that knowledge rather
than power was the goal. We would point out to the reader
that a thorough investigation of Tantric history and tradition shows that there is also a history of Black Magick,
famous Black Magicians, sorcery, and other things that
don't mesh with the Western fantasy of what Buddhism is.
This is commensurate with the idea that the accomplished

Tantric, whether Buddhist or Hindu is "beyond good and evil."

The Tantric practitioner makes choices consciously. Further, his morality is not the morality of the common herd. It is esoteric not exoteric and, as an autonomous being, he makes his own choices for his own reasons.

The goals of Hindu Tantrism, on the other hand, are much closer to the Western goals of Occultism and self-development. There are several reasons for this. First of all, it acknowledges the existence of the "Atman" (or soul) which Buddhism does not consider. Also India, unlike Tibet, suffered repeated invasions and attacks by Islamic invaders who were horrified by what they found in Universities that taught Tantric science.

As a result, the exoteric (i.e., socially accepted branch of Tantrism) disappeared in India and what we are left with is an almost entirely esoteric and secret tradition very much like the tradition of Black Magick and Satanism in Europe.

The goal of Bengali Tantrism is the development of power as well as knowledge. All societies want to prevent this in the individual unless, of course, the individual happens to be born into a certain situation (caste). The situation varies according to the culture but it is usually one of family wealth and power.

48

How can we De-Trance ourselves by using Tantra?

Dr. Charles Tart made a reputation for himself early in his career with experiments involving both drugs and hypnosis. He is one of the premier experts on trance in the United States. He is also one of the most famous American psychic researchers. He has commented extensively on "consensus trance".

Anyone who studies hypnosis seriously, which unfortunately excludes most occultists and most psychologists, will find that hypnosis itself, although there are certain bizarre phenomena involved with it in some instances, under most circumstances is quite ordinary.

If one is trapped in a situation that they can't leave for hours on end, day after day after day, like normal life in business and in school, and the same verbal signals are endlessly repeated, this is hypnosis in operation. This means that hypnosis is typical of all learning and all human programming.

Among professional hypnotherapists in this century there is an axiomatic saying that is used to dispel the average person's fear of hypnosis. We are sure that anyone who has read about it has read this stated as a fact: "No one can be hypnotized into doing anything they wouldn't ordinarily be willing to do." We will put ourselves on the line and say historically this is absolutely a lie. All one has to do is substitute the circumstances and context in which an act will take place and you can elicit *any* behavior.

There are a number of clinical and non-clinical situations where people have been made to do exactly that. And we would point out that *you do not have to know you* are being hypnotized in order for the act to be accomplished. Dr. Hyatt once put a woman under, in a restaurant in front of 50 strangers while all the time she protested. When she woke up 5 minutes latter, everyone was laughing because she talked like a baby during her trance.

We know of at least one criminal case in Europe where one man was hypnotized into committing murder. In a court of law, with medical experts on hand, it was concluded by both judge and jury that the hypnotist was guilty of murder and got the death penalty.

From what we know of the facts of the case this was entirely appropriate. The man involved as a "tool" was a deeply susceptible subject with no criminal history or conviction yet he was hypnotized (some would be more comfortable with the term "brainwashed") into committing murder and then forgetting it. He was made the fall guy, to be arrested by the police, presumably with the idea that he would be considered a crazy man.

This kind of case is often ignored by modern hypnotherapists, largely due to an ignorance of history and the desire to sell their product. This is understandable because the fears of hypnosis in our culture are still considerable. This is ironic since most people are hypnotized throughout their lives.

While generally speaking, it *is* true that the average person cannot be hypnotized into doing something they would not ordinarily do, there are exceptions.

Dr. Charles Tart, in his examination of the Gurdjieff system of self-development, points this out.

He says that there is an alternate theory which he finds, in his words, rather "sinister" and we agree with him. His idea is this: Any talented hypnotist with a susceptible patient, especially a long-term patient, can leave the post-hypnotic suggestion that no other person but the therapist can put the subject in a trance or make a suggestion to him.

From Dr. Tart's point of view the greatest hypnotist we have to deal with is so-called society as a whole: In other words, those institutions and persons who create consensus trance. (In case anyone doubts this, look into the life of Adolph Hitler.)

In Tart's view just such a suggestion is constantly made to us from the time we are old enough to talk. In other words; the culture is the hypnotist that makes the suggestion to us that no other hypnotist can make a suggestion that will have any real or lasting effect. Hence, many hypnotherapists use the phrase *de-hypnotizing* instead of hypnotizing.

We've been belaboring the concept of hypnosis because it is one of the most powerful forces and techniques that human beings have.

One of the first techniques the real hypnotist is taught is not to hypnotize but to de-hypnotize. Remember that. We do not want to start off by hypnotizing. We want to start off by de-hypnotizing. And in a metaphorical sense forgetting language, forgetting history, forgetting notions of analogy and complete correspondence between concepts.

The first thing we want to do is de-hypnotize (break set). How come? To de-hypnotize is to create freedom to hypnotize yourself. The word "hypnosis" is itself a rather pathetic word. And has been stigmatized over the centuries to such an extent that normal human beings have such fear or contempt.

For example, once we were at a restaurant where we were informed that a person was bragging that her will was so strong that no one could hypnotize her.

Within three minutes she was in a deep hypnotic trance in public. We then deliberately and abruptly woke her up with full memory and she was horrified that somebody could "control" her.

We are hypnotized by the term hypnosis. You can generate forty different reactions in a room from forty different people about the word hypnosis ranging anywhere from fraud/fake, evil/good, etc.

To de-hypnotize is the first thing that must be done in order for re-programming or a new hypnotic trance to take place. People are so hypnotized by their culture and their routines and by common stimuli that most people are not allowed to have more than 3 weeks vacation, simply because it will interfere with their work and consumer trance.

And, of course, breaking trance is de-hypnotizing. And de-hypnotizing is dangerous. For whom? For those who want you to be in a specific set of trances. No specific set of trances is perfect. In other words, there are going to be leaks in the pipe, if we want to use an hydraulic analogy. Pipes are going to break a little here and bulge a little bit there and that is what social institutions are established for.

So the idea is that society is nothing more than mass hypnosis. Tantra and techniques like Black Magick are really attempts to de-hypnotize.

That's why there are so many "problems" with it. The "scare" stories surrounding Magick, mind-control techniques and even Hatha Yoga, reflect the culture's fear of any individual or group that successfully breaks the common trance and disrupts the common consumption and production patterns.

49

How do we break the effect the words of others have on us?

One of the tenets of Tantra is that people are locked in what is called "samsara"—in delusion, in hallucination, in dream. The majority of human beings, especially those living in a tightly packed environment in a regimented situation are literally living in a dream. We call it a nightmare.

Words mean more to most people, and have more reality, than actual physical events. Symbols mean more to them than their own well-being. People can be manipulated with code words, code phrases, magical incantations if you will. If you have worked in a large office environment who of you have not heard the phrase, "Well, Mr. Smith, we're not sure you're a team player."

This has two effects. First of all the use of the word "we" indicates you have offended the tribe. The tribe has turned against you and you are about to become an outcast. And "not being a team player" suggests an assumption (which most people will go along with) that they "ought" to be a team player.

The first reaction for most people in that situation is to apologize. "Gosh, I'm sorry. I didn't mean to give that impression."

If anybody has a memory, they will recall the so-called O.J. Simpson trial. The purpose of the prosecution and the purpose of the defense is not to present evidence but to present *images* and *symbols* that will hypnotize the jury.

People will say, "My God, people are not objective?" Jurors come to a trial already with a hypnotic set. The purpose of both sides—the so-called adversary system that used in the United States—is to swing the jury through the process of hypnosis by taking a set of tacit assumptions and turning it into a fact.

Dr. Hyatt's doctoral dissertation was based on the study of the process of swaying juries by using clothes, beauty, and so forth to affect the response of the jurors to the evidence being presented by the witnesses.

Whether Mr. Simpson is responsible for the deaths of these two people or not will probably never be known.

All that will be known is how well each side was capable of using tentative, probable information to hypnotize the jurors to come up with a "reasonable" idea or value as to whether or not Mr. Simpson is guilty.

The facts are, there are no facts, at all. You look at the DNA analysis, for example and there are rules that have to be followed. Sampling rules—all sorts of very complex rules. Complexity is the ground for deep trance. The mind wants to escape and escape it does into a deep, deep trance.

The reality is that the only thing we are doing here is talking about a form of cultism. We're going to take these 12 jurors and turn them into a cult. We're going to turn them into a religious sect to determine truths.

People want to talk about reality as if it existed independent of people and their brains. Actuality is what we're simply talking about. We're talking about the human brain's reaction to information and turning that information into a hypothesis which is then turned into a dogma. If you want to get off in a criminal situation, you have to buy the best hypnotists available. To our knowledge very few people have said that But in actuality lawyers are hypnotists. And they will take bits of information (that is, small "t" truth), and then change the small "t" to a big "T"

50

*How safe are these practices and should I be analyzed
before I begin?*

Many Tantric practices are safe. Others, however, are
designed to make you anxious and fearful. In fact, that is
how and why they work. You might say, real change is a
"Course In Terror."

However like any program of self-change or self-development there are real *social* dangers.

Most psychologists would think you mad if you came to
them to be "cleared" out before beginning the process of
self-willed transformation. A teacher who is disciplined and
lacks a sense of social morality (but is socially aware) is the
best choice. This is not a joke, we mean this in all serious-
ness.

Spontaneous 'etheric' body, psychological and psychic
experiences—some of them very good, some of them very
bad—can be very shocking and painful.

However, what we want to focus on is a social issue.

When you seriously begin to practice, your interests will
change, your desires will change and you may even lose
interest in long-standing relationships. This is a great danger because people are nosy and like to "help" those who
get out of line. How many people are in the nut house today
because they were following their own path and spend too
much time talking about it to friends and families?

People will notice certain significant differences in the
new "you." This could effect your job, your marriage and a
host of other situations.

Many may find these differences threatening while others will find them attractive. You may attract a whole new set of friends, get a better job, and the like.

Some people might even recognize that you are doing something for yourself that has an indirect impact on their lives. Nonetheless, you may find that you have to deal with hostilities from quarters you didn't expect and even people you consider to be virtual strangers.

There is nothing really surprising about this since most people have read this in the common variety of self-help books.

Simple things like embarking on a program of exercise or diet may affect family and marital relationships. You may find your family and friends trying to prevent your progress.

51

What about "psychic self-defense"?

This is the primary reason for secrecy in Tantra and in the Western magical tradition.

It is also one of the reasons for extensive and consistent purification.

Self-defense does not always have to do with things that are considered supernatural or paranormal.

In normal everyday conversation, psychic self-defense is highly useful and may prevent negative effects which can occur when Tantric work occasionally goes "wrong."

One of the subjects common to the occult in general, but particularly important to the Tantras and to most of the Yogas, is the question of the *subtle body* or the various subtle bodies and psychic centers.

There are a number of models for this ranging from the ancient Egyptian, to the modern Hindu, to the Tantric. We'll name some of them and describe the Chakra system without the unnecessary Hindu phrases that can be found in any book on Yoga.

An envelope of energy, as yet unidentified by Western science, surrounds the human body. (Some laboratory researchers have only gone so far as to say that they have observed this envelope. In general, however, there is little sympathy in Western Medicine for the subtle body.)

Eastern Practitioners, going back thousands of years, and modern Indian medical professionals insist that this envelope exists. And that it is as complex as the physical human body itself.

This "aura," as it is commonly called, exists in layers. We are sure many readers will have seen drawings with bands of color representing various states of health and emotion in the body. One of the authors had a rather startling experience in a University Extension class on Psychic research. An exercise was arranged in which the bulk of the group would relax and attempt to see the aura of a subject seated on a well-lit stage. Within five minutes, the person was surrounded by bands of color extending about three feet from her body. About a third of the audience saw this clearly, the rest seeing a colorless cloud or absolutely nothing.

Some trainees in deep-tissue massage and similar body work have also experienced this unexpected result. This aura is divided into what are considered "subtle bodies." The number of bodies or souls that are considered to exist, that split apart after death and go their own way after death range from 3 to 7 depending on tradition.

The Kahunas in Hawaii believe in a tri-partite soul, each of which has it's own individual existence and splits apart after death so that a human being isn't really a single unit. While there may be a tradition of believing in a form of reincarnation in Hawaii or the transmigration of souls it's not done in a linear fashion and is rather closer to the Tibetan model than the Hindu model.

For those who are unaware of it, the Hindu model was Christianized by Annie Besant after the death of Madame Blavatsky when she became the head of the Theosophical society at the turn of the century.

Connected with this is the so-called three mind model which is particularly important in some forms of transpersonal psychology and in some forms of Magick. This is particularly popular in the West because it seems to link up with the model of the three brains.

The most primitive brain is called the reptile brain. The more complex brain, which operates most of our behavior is called the mammal brain. And the large new brain, is according to some theorists, the source of some transpersonal experience, psychic power, and the mental states described by the yogis and the magicians of the past.

How accurate any of this is in the literal sense we have no idea. We find that we have to be suspicious of making any flat statements about this ourselves, or believing any such statements made by anyone else, because there is so much cultural influence involved.

It is easy for the Westerner to believe in the three brain model because it makes the whole thing sound scientific. Make no mistake, while what we are writing about in this book is *technology,* it is *not* scientific and *cannot be* scientific.

So don't be deceived when this sort of thing is "scientized" or psychologized—or as, some Jungians have attempted to do, turn it into a metaphor—because the Kundalini experience is none of these.

52

*Can you give some examples of Kundalini phenomena,
and are there Western methods of dealing with it?*

Yes. The work of the pioneer psychiatrist Wilhelm Reich.
In the West, he was the person who came closest to analyzing the Kundalini experience in clinical terms. For his
work, the culture hounded him to his death under the guise
of protecting the public. (It seems that the preoccupation
with "safety" is always more important than the truth.)

It should be emphasized Reich was philosophically an
atheist which is what makes his work so much more interesting.

He claims to have seen, as have many others, the various
forms "of the Force." He claims to have seen "something"
floating through the air, coursing through bodies. A phenomena *similar* to Kundalini?

I (Dr. Hyatt) have often seen manifestations of this
"force" over the last thirty years in the practice of psychotherapy, ceremonial Magick, meditation and trance experiments. I do not believe that these were hallucinations or
problems with my eyes. They were very solid and bright
and behaved in ways unlike that of reflected light or "spots
before my eyes."

I firmly believe that Reich had some form of experience
that gave him this knowledge. Some have speculated that
he studied some forms of Tantra Yoga before he developed
his therapy and his theory.

Reich called these so-called auras "orgone energy." We
don't know what it *is*. It's a word Reich made up in order to

scientize what may really have been mystical experiences that his patients were having.

These were like waves of visible energy, floating over and through their body. Muscles would move and jerk in strange patterns much like the so-called snake of Kundalini.

Since Reich had great contempt for religion (he considered it one of the greatest evils—he saw it destroying man's pure bio-energetic/bio-sexual nature and thus his mind), he attempted to create a scientific model to explain what the Hindus and other groups have seen for many centuries. So he attempted to scientize it in order to make it acceptable to the public and the scientific community.

Reich attempted to develop a form of therapy around the idea of "orgone energy." He called it "Orgone Therapy."

Many people have had extensive experiences with this type of work. I'm more inclined to call it Kundalini Therapy rather than Orgone Therapy.

I (Hyatt) was lucky enough to work with Dr. Regardie for many years—including approximately three and a half years in training. Dr. Regardie, as many of you know, developed the powerful and well-known Middle Pillar technique. He also used some of the techniques of Wilhelm Reich. Together, he and I combined these practices into what we called the "Kundalini work."

In the course of his therapy practice, Regardie would charge himself with the Middle Pillar technique. He then focused the energy into his hands and placed them on "blocked" (sometimes called "armored") parts of the body of his patients. This armor held back the Kundalini (or the natural snake wave) from moving throughout the body and liberating the person from his strictures.

The theory is very simple. There are "blocks" in the body that oppose the normal flow of bio-electrical energies and prevent real orgasm.

Reich was very clear in differentiating between an ejaculation in the normal sense of the word and full orgasm in which the entire body goes into waves. In a "Reichian" orgasm, the muscles develop a wave pattern and then turn into a "full-body ejaculation."

Now many of you may think that you have had such an experience but let me assure you: there are very few people alive today who have had that type of orgasm. And, most people would not want to try to develop the ability to do that on their own because it would scare the living hell out of them. By controlling sexuality and reducing it to what we normally call orgasm, society can control the individual's sense of power and freedom. Society does this to prevent individuals from employing the proper use of sex to gain powers of self-control, relaxation, and focus and instead, allow normal people to think they really have these powers. These beliefs are just nothing more than hypnotic trances that the robots are in. (Much like the vote.)

By breaking down body armor using the specific techniques we developed, Regardie created in people the ability to have psychic powers which they never had before.

Reich would not approve of this because he discounted Magick and Religion. For Reich, the entire orgasmic process was orgone-psycho-physiological.

Reich was arrested and died in prison from a heart attack (a broken heart; in one sense). He had developed the Orgone accumulator, which in his mind accumulated energy which could be passed to the occupant of the accumulator to help break down the blocks which prevented the full orgasmic reflex. (As an interesting aside during the height of psychical research sponsored by the USSR, Psychic accumulators similar in function to Reich's were developed and "proven" to work in laboratory conditions.)

We must remind the reader that 99% of people have *not* had a full orgasmic reflex. They've had "sneezes." *True* orgasm, through the Kundalini energy, create a feeling of union with the entire universe. Some, like Dr. Hyatt, have suggested that true orgasm produces a neucoid-magnetic resonance of the individual with the planet which in turn allows the psychic integration of the planet with the entire universe.

In other words, *once the true neucoid-Kundalini process begins to flow, the person has a mystico-communion—orgasmic telepathy—with the whole world.*

We have experienced other types of neucoid-Kundalini phenomena ourselves. For example, after I (Dr. Hyatt) had a training session with Regardie, I would go out and do what I had to do and all of a sudden, out of nowhere, I would start seeing things, mostly bluish kinds of light, where you wouldn't expect to see it. I saw this energy flowing all around me. The reason that happened was that I was "loose" enough to be in contact. This attests to the power of these techniques.

In the normal person, the body shields against the orgasmic flow—yet the universe is in a constant orgasm. If you were not armored, you would be participating in this cosmic orgasm all the time. For most people this would be quite disturbing.

One of my best friends for many years (who I admire greatly to this day) had a hard time dealing with these experiences.

He held two Master's degrees; one in the hard sciences and the other in psychology, and a Doctorate of Chiropractic. He was a rationalist in the true meaning of the word. For him to believe in this form of orgasmic energy seemed ludicrous.

I convinced him to go through a number of sessions with me. He trusted me enough to know that I would not try to brainwash him into believing anything.

And then he started experiencing these things himself. He was shocked because this totally violated his rational point of view. He attempted to understand it. In fact, he went through a five year period of training with Dr. Regardie and experienced many of the things Mr. Black and I are talking about.

Because the crossover between the Kundalini experience and the work Reich developed is so important and so close in many ways, it is worth a student's time to experience at least a dozen sessions or so with a person well-qualified and open to such ideas. This does not necessarily mean a psychotherapist. In fact, most psychotherapists would not be a good choice.

One of the experiments that Mr. Black and I did was to use a combination of Kundalini therapy and hypnosis to open Mr. Black up further. We expected to receive psychic information (which he did) and our experiments proved to be highly reliable.

If you intend to employ these techniques in a practical way, you must be very cautious. For example, if you are in a relationship and you start to have strange sexual experiences with your mate, you may find them leaving you. Because you are "attacking" them—not in any deliberate way, but you are attacking the "body shield," which is their anxiety control device.

Society has developed the body shield to make you a conformist, a functional idiot—no matter how rebellious you think you are. As your shield breaks down, those around you will feel the effects of the energy you release into the environment. Most people around you experience this as "psychic pollution" which subtly attacks *their* shields and makes them feel anxiety. They will then become hostile to you.

It is important to realize is that as shields break down anxiety is the prime signal that the process is working. You'll have to develop many ways of dealing with anxiety in many forms you've never thought existed. There are all different kinds of anxiety, some of which are much more horrifying when the body shields are breaking down—particularly in a relatively uncontrolled fashion. You may begin to lose many relationships and at the same time you will begin to gain some new ones. You become like a neucoid magnet, attracting and repelling many forces.

The neucoid power travels up a "channel" which may or may not be physical. While traveling it can stop at any of the neucoid centers, which some believe roughly correspond to the seven Chakras. This can produce unexpected ecstatic or violent bodily sensations.

I (Jason Black) described my first Kundalini experience as resulting from a magical experiment I did (see *Pacts with the Devil,* New Falcon Publications).

I had been acting as a medium for a group and was already adept at self-induced trances. I was sitting in a chair, repeating the experiment at home when a wave of ecstasy started moving from the bottom of my feet all through my body. I'm not entirely sure how long this particular part of the experience lasted. It could have been anywhere from 15 to 30 minutes. But for three days I was filled with so much energy that the people at work asked me a few times if I was on speed. I was not. My face was flushed, I was giggling, I was rushing all around the place. The physical work I was supposed to do was done in a flash and it went on unabated. As pleasant as this sounds, I started to become very worried. Eventually it faded away. (New experiences usually go in waves of good and then a period I would call hibernation.)

But Kundalini and the various forces of the body, including forces which are not popular concepts in Jungian psychology or Magick in Western thought, give every impression of being outside yourself. That is, the classic attack of forces from beyond. Spiritual forces, psychic forces, whatever you want to call them. This can be very frightening. As such, the practitioner must always be aware that having these experiences can discourage one from continuing the work.

The experience will go away, and you will find you have made progress. It should also be pointed out that bad feelings are often signs of progress. Using a locker room analogy, whenever anyone begins a period of vigorous exercise, especially weightlifting, there is a period when one experiences toxicity.

When you first begin to exercise, various toxins accumulated in the fat in your body are released into the body and make you feel bad. This release can continue for several weeks. After this passes you begin to feel wonderful after exercise.

One supposition is that in some of these experiences you are opening areas of "psychic infection" (i.e., negativity that is stored in the psyche—and by the psyche we are referring to the Greek concept rather than the psychological idea).

This is the idea of mind as a field rather than a function of the brain. And the field extends throughout your body and possibly beyond it. On the other hand, there are other experiences where you have the feeling of being attacked from forces outside. If you talk about this to people who haven't had similar experiences you make yourself sound paranoid and crazy. Our advice in a situation like this is to be very careful before assuming that the attack is literally coming from outside, especially if you think it is from another person; otherwise you can make terrible social blunders.

In societies where witchcraft and sorcery are openly practiced (e.g., aboriginal societies where shamanism is still practiced), the attitude is that a spell is being cast upon you even if the person casting it is *unaware* that he is casting it. This, from a modern point of view, is paranoid. But those of you familiar with psychic research may see that it's not necessarily an unwarranted idea.

In any event, if you are having such an experience, treat the experience seriously and perform a ritual of protection for yourself. Operate under the assumption that the force is real—it is real for you if you are experiencing it—but don't judge it, don't call yourself crazy and don't assume other people and other things are attacking you simply because of the experience until you have further information. But the practitioner should be warned that these experiences do occur and they often occur for no reason that can be readily seen.

Dr. Regardie was very clear that "psychiatric symptoms" are a necessary sign that the methodology is working. However, when we talk about something like this we feel like withdrawing a bit because of the structure of our society and the medical and psychological approach to things. Because sometimes the symptoms that do break through are quite real, as in Neucoid-Kundalini therapy while the shield is dissolving. In fact, you may be *making* the symptoms real. Because you are acting strange, people are going to be acting strange toward you. It is important to realize that you can get yourself into a lot of trouble and this is one reason we suggest you move slowly and cautiously.

It can also be useful to keep a journal containing the facts and avoid interpretation.

Interpretation, as a rule, will often lead a person down the rosy path of hell, where sooner or later you start believing in theories to justify or explain away your unpleasant experiences. Much like people believe in religion or Jesus.

53

Can you suggest some experiments to deal with this issue?

The first experiment is to get a piece of white paper and a black pen or pencil. Close your eyes and starting making dots all over the paper. Make them all over the place. After a few minutes; stop, open your eyes and watch your mind try to make patterns of the dots and watch what your mind attempts to create. Watch your mind play "Connect the Dots." All of a sudden you'll see your mind say, "Ah, this is how the lines are *supposed* to go together" and you'll start drawing solid lines through *all* of the dots. You'll come up with a pattern and say, "My, God there it is. This is what these dots were *really* referring to."

Now, throw away your idea of what they were supposed to look like and try the experiment all over again.

In fact, if you make some Xerox copies and you can then use the same dots. Just start out with a different assumption or hypothesis of what the dots were supposed to look like or supposed to mean.

This is called "filling in" and was studied by the Gestalt theorists, the ability of the mind to make order out of what appears to be disorder. So in your experiments and in your techniques attempt to develop a facility of creating theories and absurdities out of random dots and you will begin to see why so many people act like idiots.

Because not only do they *not* see most of the dots, not only do they fail to see that they have selected certain dots from which they draw lines to create pictures, sooner or later they come to believe that it was the "intention" of the dots to create that particular picture. You can argue with them for the rest of your life and theirs and five more incarnations and they will not give up that belief.

What we have just described is an example of what the Tibetans see as void-as-matter and matter-as-void. This is something that used to confuse SJB greatly he accidentally read a footnote by Professor Evans Wentz in one of the Tibetan books: they simply meant the penetration of matter and mind on a psychic level. There is no word in the Tibetan language for psychic phenomena, because, for them, the world is *an example* of psychic phenomena.

The projection of meaning to lines made from random dots on a piece of paper is analogous to the projection of reality, either in terms of meaning or in terms of physical reality, from the mind of the person doing the projecting.

We will speak briefly about Karma.

Karma is not "justice." That childish notion is common among Christians in the West and among Eastern peasants it is used to keep people in line.

Karma, as Alan Watts pointed out, in its esoteric meaning is *attachment*. And this attachment is not just psychological but psychic in the paranormal sense. That is you will create or attract that which deep down you think is appropriate for you or that you deserve.

Good luck, bad luck, meeting a certain type of person will happen over and over again, until the Karma (connection) is broken. And the Buddhists, especially are concerned with breaking this connection. This can be done in a number of different ways and is quite often done violently. By "violently" we don't necessarily refer to *physical* violence, although there have been certain sects that went that far.

We mean psychological violence, psychic violence.

The Tibetan Buddhists have what they call the Chod rite which is a holdover from the Shamanic tradition in Tibet that existed before the arrival of a Tantra in the 7th Century.

In this rite the aspirant goes to a graveyard (for the Hindu this is a burning ground), where bodies are taken to a charnel ground and left for the animals to eat. So it's even more colorful than the Hindu version and when the flesh is stripped from the bones by the animals the bones are taken and jewelry is made from them. (Many of you have seen skull bowls and thigh horns that are used in rituals. Some of these items are relatively easy to buy in the United States.)

The aspirant enters the graveyard, usually at night, and induces a trance. (How this trance is induced we have never seen described specifically. Presumably because he is a trained Buddhist monk he is able to enter the trance through meditation. Yet, since this is a survival of Shamanic tradition, hallucinogenic drugs may be used.)

He lies down, sometimes in a pit, to imitate a shallow grave, and experiences demons appearing and devouring his body. Apparently this experience is so intense that every once in a while an aspirant doesn't survive.

The idea behind this is to literally destroy your previous state and put it back together. Other manifestations of this are some of the higher states of Yogic practice.

(We have experienced the state that is generally referred to as "no mind" for very brief times and, when we came out of the state found remarkable physical changes in our bodies and changes in the emotional state of our minds.)

The idea is that when they enter this state of mind, they cease to exist on a psychic level and then they reintegrate themselves on a higher level. This is one of the signs of progress in Tantra.

One of the more extreme and disapproved of Hindu techniques involves the act of committing actual violent crime in order to become indifferent to it.

We don't mean *hardened* to it (though that is involved as well) but the realization comes that all of the rules are arbitrary with no exception and are to be transcended. (Here you might reflect upon the analogy of the connected dots.)

Any aspirant who is to reach full development as an Adept must realize this at the very core of his being so that any choice he makes in action or thought or life is made fully on his own. Thus all choice is fully appropriate to the circumstances. This attitude bothers some people because it sometimes involves "strange" practices as well as attitudes toward the community, neighbors and friends which people find frightening, since they are uncontrolled by cultural taboos.

We have found that the very fact that we have disavowed Christianity and have embraced active occult activities has occasionally targeted us from unexpected sources. People we hardly know have shown a great deal of hostility and active fear and horror.

The general idea is that if "he doesn't believe as I do or if he doesn't believe in these ideals (pick a norm, pick an ideal, it doesn't matter) he's *capable of anything.*"

In a positive sense, that is the goal. To be capable of anything in a positive sense—positive at any given time, the appropriate action to the appropriate circumstance. However, people bound up in hypnosis, in trance, say, "If he doesn't believe in [you fill in the blank]..." and that usually ends up in accusations of Satanism or whatever the cultural Taboo of the hour considers "evil."

That means they think you are capable of doing any crime and doing it to them. It's also an act of extreme jealousy because the majority of people are not happy with their lives and are trapped in an endless round of habit until they're put six feet under or they retire and completely lose their minds through boredom.

54

What is the difference between humans and other animals?

To illustrate, we will relate a scene from the book *Dune* by Frank Herbert.

This book (which was also produced as a movie of the same name) is a fictional account with a great deal of authentic Tantric material in terms of attitudes, goals and practices. (In SJB's opinion, *Dune* is one of the best pieces of fiction ever written on the subject; it was written in the form of science fiction which frees it from any cultural baggage.)

In one of the early scenes, the son of Duke Atreides—who is later to become the Kwisatz Haderach, the Messianic figure on the planet *Dune*—is awakened from a sound sleep by an old woman, a member of the mystical Order called Bene Gesserit, who says she is going to give him a test to see if he's human.

She places his hand in a box that interfaces directly with his nervous system. In a short time he begins to feel painful sensations, as if his hand is being burned and the flesh is peeling away from his bones.

She holds a poison needle against his neck and states that if he makes the slightest move to escape, she'll kill him.

She tells him this very clearly.

And she means it.

The message is clear: if you have the control and awareness to resist the desire to run, then you have shown yourself to be a human being.

Otherwise you are an animal and you deserve to die.

He passes the test and the story proceeds.

This story relates a typically Tantric view. She was saying to him that this is an initiation: you're either going to prove you have the wherewithal and the abilities to be a human being or you are an animal and I'll kill you like an animal.

Among the Hindu Tantrics there is a word and a phrase. The word is "Pashu" and the phrase "Pashu Innana." Pashu means "animal" or "uninitiated" and Pashu Innana is usually translated as "uninitiated beast." This may sound like the sort of insult any religion or cult gives to an individual who doesn't belong to it. (Christianity and Islam are notorious for this.)

In fact, the psychology of Tantra indicates they are speaking literally. The person who is not initiated, the person who does not have the wherewithal to develop himself beyond the expectations of society or in spite of those expectations, is *literally*—not figuratively—an animal.

He is no more intelligent or useful to the world or to himself than a talking dog. (It might be noted that, in recent years, zoologists have taught both chimpanzees and gorillas to speak English using sign language or electronic means at the level of a well-developed child.)

It's extremely dangerous on a personal level, especially if you have involved yourself in a program of self-development and change, to think of the humans you pass on the streets as people at all.

What you're dealing with is a cluster of stimulus-response behaviors that is about as dangerous as a trained rattlesnake.

This can be particularly seen in any time of political trouble when the lower middle classes—the least intelligent large group in any society—become dangerous and physically violent when it becomes clear that they are not as important as they were told by Church and State and Mommie and Daddy: that they are mere cogs in a wheel that can be exchanged at a moment's notice by their higher-ups.

Currently in the United States there is a phenomenon called the "angry white male." There's also the angry black male and a host of other angry males. What one political commentator said is that what they are really talking about is the angry blue collar male.

We believe this quite correct. People who really are powerless on a political and economic level and don't have any intellectual depth, are really no more than a cluster of stimulus-response patterns who are outraged when they see themselves as truly worthless.

They see themselves as victims. They see themselves as robbed. And there must be a scapegoat. And this is where they become the tools of unscrupulous politicians or power-mongers.

They blame Communists, Nazis or become Communists or Nazis, they blame Jews, they blame Homosexuals, they blame Blacks, they blame Satanists. A host of things. Anything that makes them a victim and therefore a potential hero by resisting. This kind of mentality causes physical violence. It causes an increase in crime in quarters where crime is not normally committed.

It is a truly dangerous situation. This is why we say that such people are not to be trusted if you are pursuing a program of self-development. These are, in the words of the Hindus, Pashu. These are people so bound up by limited intellectual capacity combined with habits of thought and activity that they are unable to change. This group didn't even know that there were dots to connect, they are about as friendly and helpful as a herd of stampeding elephants.

This becomes particularly true when this group of people becomes threatened at particular levels of identity which are tied to certain buzz symbols ("the house"), or certain social concepts ("the family"), and such forms of superiority as "decent," "Christian," and "law abiding."

As we go through our next cultural change, you will see that *these* people will become the most interesting group of all because those in the middle class are literally incompetent.

When *their* status is removed, their economic power is removed All they're going to do is cry.

The blue collar male, on the other hand are going to be extremely dangerous because their whole sense of worth is contradicted by the images they see on TV.

They hold their pathetic egos together, like the Nazis, by a superiority based on nothingness. Then, finally they are even robbed of their "decent" illusion.

55

What is the most fundamental problem involved in group work?

Among the Hindu Tantrics there is a word and a phrase. The word is "Pashu" and the phrase is "Pashu Innana." Pashu means "animal" or "uninitiated" and Pashu Innana is usually translated as "uninitiated beast." The Pashu is conceived as a herd animal and is subject to a pitfall that is a result of religious or occult symbolism, namely, idealism in its worst sense.

We are not referring to a person's doing the very best he can in a certain situation or developing himself in a way that will improve his lot, or his life, or his abilities.

We are talking about *group* idealism and *political* idealism at the same level that we speak of sentimentality as false emotion.

We have met a number of people in religion and in so-called occult Orders who believe that they are going to change the world or that they've inherited the earth or that they are going to create the new man.

All of this is generally spoken of against a background of truly overwhelming mediocrity.

This kind of intellectual compensation behavior is one of the things that weeds out people most frequently and most thoroughly in any kind of self-development that involves a group.

One of the most profound and interesting qualities that involves the idea of idealism is the belief that ideas are more real than actuality.

This form of philosophy, more often than not, acts as a tranquilizer, a shot of whiskey, a pain pill, etc. because the individual cannot deal with the actualities of existence. And most of us cannot really deal with this issue in a painless way. So we like to make ourselves feel better. It's sort of a form of Medicare from birth. Or, if you would, like belonging to certain peer groups.

We try to make ourselves feel better by providing ourselves with ideas that attempt to substitute for the boredom, the loneliness, the emptiness, the day-to-day experience and numbness of our normal lives.

People spend a lot of time developing theories and philosophies about so-called "ideas" simply as a form of mental entertainment (some might call it masturbation), because it provides them with a sense of relief from the monotony, the inevitability, the aging, the pain, the suffering of daily life.

Holidays often serve the same purpose. One technique we have learned is to make your own Holidays. Learn how to make your own celebrations.

In any discussion of evolution or initiatory steps we will use a number of words and ideas; these should be absorbed broadly. You can forget the words themselves so long as you do not forget the concept. One of the principle goals of becoming a Tantric adept in the Bengali tradition is to develop the concept of Siddi, to become a Sidda: that is, a Saint with power.

From the European point of view this would be a Magician: an adept with power, one who has psychic, physical or intellectual powers beyond the norm. This is often considered to be beneath consideration by some non-Tantric Buddhists. (However we should point out that the Tantric Buddhists have, as their earliest Saints, the Siddas they inherited from the Bengali.)

So there is a bit of a double standard there. In the Hindu system the beginning point for any person who is considered eligible for development is called Vira.

This idea does not describe an ordinary man, but rather a man with potential. A man with power. Possibly a genius—though probably not.—but a man with the potential for genius, the potential for development.

This is the person who first enters into Tantric study and is accepted by the Guru.

In the West, if a Guru is not available, often the candidate's own spirit is sufficient for creating an Astral guide or creating the correct circumstances. Often this is called the Holy Guardian Angel.

Such a candidate is a person with strong will, with high ambitions, and with qualities outside the norm which may or may not be considered social eccentricity. These qualities can be athletic, mental, spiritual, sexual, even extreme beauty provided they are combined in such a way that they can be utilized for the advancement of the organism. By "organism" we mean the mental, spiritual and physical machine all together as a unit.

In all of the Tantras—especially the Bengali Tantras—there is still the concept of right-hand and left-hand paths.

Some occultists who were scared silly by what they read about the Tantras in various Westernized writings equated the left-hand path with evil, the Christian Devil.

Tantra, in it's left-hand form, is considered evil especially by anyone who is Orthodox in the Christian sense.

56

*What does Tantra say about the arbitrary nature of all
rules?*

This includes *all* rules of morality. This does not necessarily mean that one goes around breaking rules simply as
an act of defiance, but that one does not suffer from those
rules—or fears of hell, or any such nonsense—simply
because the rules exist and you're told to follow them.

Robert Lindner, Ph.D., in his book *Prescription for
Rebellion* (1952), discussed the whole notion of rebellion.
For example, there is the idea of defiance. At its highest
level, defiance is merely a tool for a specific purpose and
not a virtue in itself.

However, for an adolescent, defiance is not just a technique. It's a methodology of growth and development. And,
as such, defiance is essential to the society that loathes it.

In other words, without defiance there would not be a
society. Society requires new blood and fresh ideas which,
in one form or another, are utilized by the system for its
own diabolic purposes.

There are many more good masters than there are good
students and you can figure out the mathematics of that
yourself. But, as a rule, a good student has to be made.
Normally a good student (whether in college, high school,
or grammar school) is compliant and obedient and knows
how to follow instructions.

In a certain sense, knowing how to follow instructions
and perform activities within a Tantric training system are
essential. But these are not done by rote or for social training. Nor are they done for a position in a future life so that

when you're 25 years old you can afford to have one wife or one husband, three children and two and a half cars in your garage.

Obedience is a useful technique much as defiance is a useful technique. But it is very clear that rebellion (which can be considered a form of defiance), is biologically essential for a newer organism to take its place in society and gain a sense of its own individual advancement.

True defiance or true rebellion—or, for that matter, true obedience—are essential to take control, or develop control over your own life and create your own sense of identity apart from the crowd.

To talk about being apart from the crowd creates a number of contradictions. One is always implying some form of positive or negative valence. These are called "juxtapositions." We juxtapose supposedly contradictory things, one thing against another. These are just maneuvers and are not realities. For example, there is no such thing as a complete difference between night and day. The amount of light constantly changes throughout the day and the amount of "darkness" constantly changes throughout the night. They are continuous—they are not real opposites.

People almost always speak in terms of "points of view" and usually there are only two. And it is all very simplex and very interesting and most people spend their lives suffering in this form of herd instinct.

It reduces their anxieties much as their idealism does. Their religious beliefs, their family holidays, their social gatherings, their parties, their Saturday night, their Sunday brunch. All of these routines are simply methods of getting through life and to the grave without having lived.

Tantra is designed to do the exact opposite.

57

What are the steps of Tantric initiation?

The Vira (a man with potential, an exceptional man) is often a troublemaker and rebel as a youth or even as an adult. For example, many people who become famous as writers, artists, rock stars or politicians (but *that* hardly ever applies) were once considered stupid or unmanageable or even mentally ill when they were children.

They were often asked, "Why can't you be like everyone else?"

The real goal of the machine, as exemplified by public school systems all over the world, is to produce the average shopkeeper. Most "good students" that we've encountered, later on become nice, moderately successful insurance salesmen, housing developers, managers of large department stores—something of that order. In other words they were manufactured goods. There are a number of famous people who, if you investigated their backgrounds, were filled with trouble. This is really remarkable and a true indication of what we are talking about.

We are *not* suggesting, however, that every social misfit on the street is an advanced Adept—or even an initate. Most who make such claims simply want to find an excuse to feel better about themselves.

The fundamentalist churches of America, as well as various esoteric and splinter religious groups, are filled with such people. They are absolutely *not* what we are talking about here.

These people are just more drones and just a part of the herd—or sometimes a splinter of the herd which has been rejected by the larger group.

The next step up in our very brief definition of initiation is, in Hindu terms, the Kala. In Bengali Tantra the Kala is the person who has actually taken the step to enter a brotherhood, accept a Guru and take the beginning steps to development.

Many in the West operate without a teacher, with only the information he can glean and with the guidance of his own instincts. So, for this purpose, we might define the Kala as anyone who has started on the path, physically, literally, with intention; started doing the work in a committed way and has begun experiencing the results.

Moving on to the next level, we might speak of a person who is on his way to genuine deprogramming, the deprogramming of the psycho-social chains that he has been bound with. This person will, bit by bit, begin to experience not only an increase in his personal abilities but also a number of the negative effects.

The shock of realizing that people around him—his peers—are little more than robots or cattle will be an unpleasant revelation.

He will experience the shock of disassociation and most likely the disavowal of the religious and social principles he was raised to cherish.

He will experience the shock of psychic phenomena— from dreams to premonitions to actual apparitions. While he is still balancing the values and ideas of reality he was raised with against his new experiences, he may very well question his sanity.

There is no better response.

There is absolutely nothing wrong with this. We worry about people who don't question their sanity when they first begin to experience these things.

People who never question what they experience or its validity often become religious fanatics or consider themselves to be prophets and cease their progress altogether.

The work has been wasted.

On the other hand, the person on the path gradually becomes more and more extreme in his practices and more and more committed to his practices.

The Kala ultimately is on his way to becoming a Sidda: someone who has power. This power may be charismatic or psychic. Many experience remarkable changes in their abilities, have prophetic dreams, influence things around them, make changes in their physical bodies and their habits without following the ordinary logical/linear course taught in our culture.

58

What are some modern Tantric techniques that I can use every day to help me change?

In his remarkable book, *Prometheus Rising* (New Falcon Publications, 1984), Robert Anton Wilson suggests an exercise: "Be a Nazi for a day."

(Imagine you are on television and suggest to all the members of our so-called culture to be a Nazi for a day. It might be very difficult for them because they are not already Nazis. If they are Nazis *at all,* most of them are Nazis for a lifetime.)

But the point should be very clear: learn how to take on different dogmas, different philosophies, believe in them fully and act them out—within the limits of the law, of course—and help yourself break your own label and your own dogma. Each of us is a dogma, each is a philosophy, in the sense that each of us is a metaphor in our own mind. In this sense we are not real.

When Dr. Wilson suggested this exercise, the publisher received a number of letters from people who were horrified with the idea that someone could recommend practicing being a Nazi for a day.

It is interesting to note that most ignored that he also suggested being a born-again Christian for a day. Here again is the juxtaposition of good and evil. Most people are only capable of thinking in a very simplex, socially contained, consensual process—that is, to be a Nazi for a day is evil and to be a born-again Christian for a day is good—because one implies destruction and one does not. Ha!

This is absurd. Born-again Christians—and Christianity itself—has murdered more people than all the Nazis in the world and, in point of fact, if you wanted to apply the word "Nazi" as commonly understood to a group of people it might best be applied to the born-again Christians.

Dr. Wilson suggests another exercise in this area: "Become a pious Roman Catholic. Explain in three pages why the Church is still infallible and holy despite Popes like Alexander VI (the Borgia Pope), and Pious XII (ally of Hitler), etc.

The simple fact is that the "Christians" are seen as good because they won their war (long ago) and the Nazis, using the *same tactics* in their struggle are evil because they lost.

In all of this, of course, Dr. Wilson's real point is easily lost. He is saying: Set your mind to something, practice it, do it, become it, and see what you experience. See what happens to you.

Another practice he suggested was to start looking for quarters on the street. This is another exercise for a day of great self-transformation. If you find yourself looking for quarters you will find more quarters. They do not magically appear. You start looking for quarters and begin to find them. This is also a fantastic demonstration of what is called the "witch hunt." You create the notion of a witch, you define it in the binary sense: us versus them. Then you will find them everywhere. No matter where you look, you will find witches.

As a method, Tantra teaches you to stand back while being deeply involved. It teaches you to live within the structure of values—or non-values—that you have created through your personal and direct experiences, from your own experiments, often with the guidance of someone who has been there before.

The purpose of the guide or guru is not as so many people in the cosmic fluff occult movement today believe; it is not to dominate you, to tell you what to think. You've already done that. Your mother and father told you that. Your teachers told you what to think. And today most people are dumb enough to believe that what they think is what *they* think. In fact people do not think at all, but rather have strings of disembodied images and associations channeled through a cultural context.

It's nothing more than a really simplex system. Human beings are fundamentally stupid. Fundamentally ignorant and fundamentally stupid. It's really two different things. Ignorant you can do something about but stupid you can't.

Most human beings are just stupid drones. The Japanese society is considered superior by many. That is, they are superior in being able to take individuals and turn them into more and better functioning 'cogs' whose value they measure by the amount of money they are able to create.

So money here is nothing more than a token of success, a measure of success. It's a dogma. Like looking for quarters and finding them. Or being a Nazi or being a born-again Christian or being a Hasidic Jew. The measure of success is always self-defined. And we are not using the word *self* in the way it's usually meant.

In the person's mind—which they often call the self—there are standards of comparison with other types. They use these mental scales to determine their position in the hierarchy of human beings.

And if they fall short of that standard which has been implanted in their brain, they become unhappy. They become unhappy and they begin to look for happiness in directions which are not considered normal. Even though they do find some happiness in these directions it is not without a price. Reactive happiness carries the price of the guilt that stands behind it.

In European philosophy the problem of deviant guilt was solved by the Marquis de Sade. He did this by affirming the absolute sovereignty of the individual above the group.

More recently, Aleister Crowley did something similar. However, his thinking has been perverted by many of his modern adherents. He said, "Do what thou wilt shall be the whole of the Law. Love is the law, love under will."

59

What comes after initiation?

Once the candidate of initiation or Adeptship has passed the point of being a mere candidate and becomes a practitioner, one of the earliest goals is to develop within the organism what is referred to in both Eastern and Western techniques as the "subtle organs."

There are so-called subtle sheaths and astral bodies which surround the person; their various functions can include pure emotion and pure intellect—which can include the receiving and processing of information from the minds of other people. However, according to both Eastern and Western thought (mostly Eastern), there are specific organs that have an existence that is more solid than imagination but more ephemeral than pure physical matter and that have to be dealt with and developed before any real progress can be made.

When these organs are dealt with in the proper manner the practitioner is able to receive material from his intuition and from other sources that he was unable to receive before—accurate and checkable information, guidance for his life.

All of these things can and do happen spontaneously in the population at large and often manifest themselves in ways depending on the cultural background of the person. For example, whether a person has had a religious background or not may affect the experience of a psychic vision (which in Tantric physiology would have something to do with the Brow Chakra). One with a religious background might assume he had a revelation from God and might go off the deep end in some way and join a fundamentalist Church, thus wasting the rest of his life as a result of a mania caused by a perfectly natural phenomena fueled by ignorance.

Two other "post-initiation" issues are Kundalini (dictionary definition: energy that lies dormant at the base of the spine until it is activated, as by the practice of yoga, and channeled upward through the chakras in the process of spiritual perfection) and the Chakras (dictionary definition: the centers of spiritual energy in the human body according to yoga philosophy).

It is very important to note that some of the phenomena caused by the so-called Kundalini experience can be very intense and can involve both emotional and physical phenomena that are both alien and unpleasant to our culture. Often, the only answer to the situation (from the points of view of both the person experiencing it and of the people around him), is to take him to a psychiatrist and put him on drug therapy.

While there is some research being conducted into the so-called Kundalini syndrome in the United States today, few people are doing it. And, unless you're familiar with the literature already, and have access to someone at the Esalen Institute, you are in very deep trouble indeed if you are ignorant about what's going on. You have been warned!

Aside from the subtle sheaths that surround the body and reflect and influence its health and mental function, there are these things called Chakras. The Chakras are wheels of light (or are visualized as wheels of light) and are placed at various points in the subtle body system.

Traditionally it is said that there are seven major Chakras. However, in some cultures where medicine acknowledges this system there are many more.

The technique of acupuncture medicine (which, after a great deal of debate—it must be thirty years or more now—was finally accepted as a legitimate medical technique even though no one can adequately explain exactly how it works) is an example of the manipulation of this energy. For the Chinese, it is described as the flow of Ki (Chi) (which is essentially the flow of Kundalini) in small invisible channels throughout the body. It should also be emphasized that these channels are said to have a semi-real, semiphysical nature.

Some doctors assume that, when the acupuncturist practices his trade, he is dealing with the central nervous system in ways unknown to the West. In fact, if one studies an acupuncture chart or a three dimensional model with the acupuncture zones marked upon it, some of the most important acupuncture points are at places where there are no nerve endings—indeed, where there is no nexus of nerves or muscles of any kind.

Broadly speaking, in Tantric technique these subtle organs are generally intended to be influenced in three ways.

First, by *magical ritual*—and we specifically use the term "magical ritual" as opposed to "religious ritual" because of the attitude and focus involved which is not so much *worshipful* but *purposeful and demanding* in regard to whatever supernatural beings are alleged to be involved.

Second, through *rhythmic breathing* and third, through *trance work* and the *mental visual stimulation* of the organs themselves. (The complex system of Hatha Yoga is also used for this purpose. A person interested in this form of Yoga can find volumes on this subject, or may seek direct guidance from Hindu practitioners.)

As stated earlier, there are seven major Chakras that theoretically tie in with Kundalini.

The theory is quite simple: the life force within the body (which is normally uncontrolled) is supposed to rise from the bottom to the top. In actual practice, and if you study the Hindu documents themselves, you'll find that a host of phenomena are involved with Kundalini and that it can spread any way through the body: bottom to top, top to bottom, from the base (Muladhara) Chakra which is usually considered to be near the anus but can even come from the bottom of the feet.

The seven Chakras are commonly placed thusly:

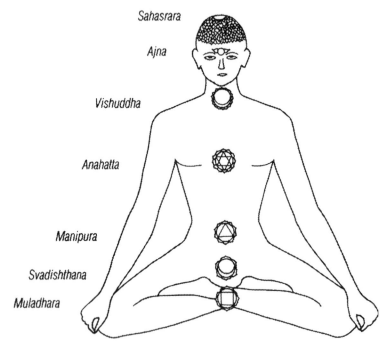

Sahasrara

Ajna

Vishuddha

Anahatta

Manipura

Svadishthana

Muladhara

The Base Chakra (Muladhara) is considered to be the seat of the potential Kundalini itself. This is where the power is stored and, in most people, this is where it remains. (Thus, in most people Kundalini functions only at its lowest level as a physical force while the higher intellectual and spiritual centers remain inert, potential and non-operational.)

In visualization work this Chakra is seen as a ball of light that extends below your buttocks, centered in the area of your rectum. The next higher Chakra would be visualized as a ball of light around the area of the genitals. Going upward again, around the area of the stomach there is another major Chakra, another ball of light. This plexus area is where the "tumo" effect begins. ("Tumo" refers to the psychic heat that is is related to Kundalini and is produced by certain meditational practices that do not have any known "trigger" and occurs regardless of the temperature you are in or the activity of your body.)

Going further up is the Heart Chakra which is supposed to stimulate major emotions: love, powers of attraction, sensitivity, even luck. (It is associated with the solar energy which, astrologically is associated with a host of good things.)

Above that is the Throat Chakra, centered right around the area where your vocal chords would be. It has to do with communication in any form. The opening of this Chakra releases tension in the throat area, including vocal tension and problems with speech.

Going upwards again we reach the Brow Chakra. This is the one most useful to psychics. It is centered right between the eyes and just above the bridge of the nose. This is also known as the 'third eye' and is associated with the God Shiva. And its power is associated with the power of destruction as is the Hindu God Shiva.

The Brow Chakra is associated with destruction in the sense that, when you bring psychic insight—including the power to increase visualization, predict the future and read minds—illusions are destroyed.

One of the points of enlightenment that occurs with work with the Brow Chakra (and can occur spontaneously with any type of Yogic practice) is, what a friend once referred to as 'endarkenment.'

Without preparation and without gradual intellectual development, one is suddenly confronted with the certainty that the people around him are robots; that the negative things—cultural hypnotism, human helplessness and addiction to human habit—come as a sudden revelation as opposed to an initiation for which one has gradually prepared.

(It is interesting to note that Dr. Israel Regardie's Middle Pillar technique has some striking similarities. Wilhelm Reich described such a the world view to be the same as a schizophrenic or as a person whose armor is dissolving.)

This can be a very damaging and a very stressful experience if it occurs without the person *being aware* that such a thing was possible.

The final, and supposedly most important Chakra of all is the Crown Chakra, centered at the top of the head (or, according to some authorities just above the top of the head). It has been pictured as a glowing White Lotus. In some highly stylized statues and pictures of the Buddha, especially in the Tibetan representations, we often see him wearing what may seem almost like a swimming cap made of little petals.

This is the iconographic representation of the complete opening of the Crown Chakra in the Buddha. It is total realization. It is total connection with the transpersonal universe which provides a way of seeing things and events which is completely non-linear and completely beyond what the average person is able to conceive. Theoretically, because of the complete change of the relation of the person to the universe, the person who has experienced this is able to produce miracles.

Probably the best description of the opening of the Kundalini all the way to the Crown Chakra was written by the Hindu Gopi Krishna in his book *Kundalini*. His description of the physical and emotional stress which can result from the sudden and unprepared for arousal of this particular force is very detailed. Any practitioner of *any* form of Yoga should take this very seriously because, whether you're attempting to arouse the Kundalini or not, doing certain techniques unknowingly or improperly can greatly affect the experience of this stress.

But don't get scared away by any of this. Having a great massage therapist can often help you overcome any minor crisis. Major disasters are few and far between and, if you begin slowly, everything should move along nicely.

The principle difficulty in dealing with the Kundalini force (or any of the life forces in general) isn't so much in *arousing* it but in *maintaining* it's arousal: maintaining its usefulness and keeping it under your control. At first it is like a wild pet.

One of Tantra's axioms is that Tantra is the quick way to achievement but it's also the dangerous way since the aspirant can fall any number of times before he achieves.

One description of Tantric practice depicts a serpent crawling up the inside of a hollow bamboo stalk. If the serpent doesn't get his chin over the opening of the top of the stalk and pull himself through, he is always in danger of falling back to the bottom and being restricted to the position in which he began.

It isn't our intention to scare people who are interested in beginning this sort of practice; in fact the benefits *far* outweigh the dangers. But, at the same time, we don't want people to walk into a practice that has certain dangers—just as physical exercise has certain dangers—and then abandon it completely at the first unpleasant experience. If you are serious, we suspect the unpleasant experiences are inevitable and simply have to be gotten past as with any other difficulty in life.

In talking about the subtle body and Kundalini, one thing is very important to both Buddhist and Hindu Tantra: the idea of positive and negative principles—the Shiva and Shakti in Hindu terms. Many erroneous things have been written about this matter. One writer recently remarked that Tantrism is goddess worship. This is simply not true. In fact, in Tantric Buddhism the notion of worshipping a God is not at all the way we think of it and they would consider the notion absurd.

On its most primitive level, to a person who has barely been initiated, it may seem to be that Tantrism *is* goddess worship. However, it should be pointed out that in Bengali Tantra in India the power force—the Kundalini, the Shakti that is attempting to be arisen—is viewed to be female. The still force—the passive force that is stimulating it to be aroused—is considered to be male.

Now, many interpret this to mean that the male force is the weaker force dominated by the Kundalini. Not so. In Hindu Tantra as in Buddhist Tantra the male force (or male figure in the iconography) is considered to be the controlling force. In the concepts of Hindu Tantra the Shakti—which is pictured as female is wild and uncontrolled—is dominated, manipulated, controlled and focused by the stillness of the male form. For example, Kali dancing on Shiva is not the *triumph* over Shiva; on the contrary Kali is doing all the work and Shiva doesn't have to do a damn thing because he's really the one who is in control.

In Tibetan Tantra it's very much the opposite. The active principle is male and the opposite principle that is used or manipulated in the iconography is female. React as you wish to the sexism involved in this. It is totally cultural and also totally irrelevant. Use what you like.

The important point is this: from the point of view of the aspirant you're uniting two aspects of yourself that are disconnected in the average person. They are considered to be opposite poles of existence. You can view them as persons. (Indeed, in India a number of Tantrics think it is safest to view it in some specific, concrete form that can be related to as a human.)

You may certainly do it in any way you wish. For example, among the Buddhists in Tibet spontaneous God forms would appear to them (the authors have also had this experience, among others). These were not necessarily temple images, but highly personal spontaneous images. This phenomena is very similar to the experiences of magicians in medieval Europe.

It's often assumed, primarily by people with their own sexual prejudices, that male aspirants always visualize females and that females always visualize males. In practice, it is often the reverse.

60

*I am more familiar with Western rituals. Can you give
me a Western ritual which has the same effect as
Tantric ritual?*

Ritual of the Demonic Spirit

This is a Shiva Shakti Western Kundalini ritual which can
be adapted either to sex acts or a symbolic Eucharist. It is a
substitute for "the five M's" of the Tantric tradition.

Its imagery is based largely on the biblical Apocalypse of
St. John and is taken from these sources:
— Chapter thirteen of the Apocalypse.
— *The Vision and the Voice* by Aleister Crowley.
— The Grimoire of Honorius.
— Portions of the traditional Latin Mass.
— Brief excerpts from the Magickal manuscripts of Dr.
John Dee.

The ritual may be performed alone or in a group. There is
a "central" section regarding an offering. This may be sexual or it may take the form of some other matter common to
both Voodoo and all Western Magick.

There follows a eucharist (which is not nearly as Christian as it looks at first glance).

The ritual deliberately utilizes images from the Apocalypse (the Beast and Babalon) as substitutes for the two
principles which must be united to arouse the kundalini
force.

If these images scare you because of childhood training,
good!

The altar may be a table with appropriate images (let your imagination and your libido run wild), or an appropriately large space on a carpeted floor, supplied with cushions, especially if the sexual aspect is to be more than symbolic. If specific beings aside from the Babylon/Beast symbology are to be evoked, their symbols or images may be placed upon the altar.

[The celebrant stands in the middle of the ritual space and recites to the four quarters of the compass]:

Conjuration of the King of the East:

I conjure and invoke thee, O powerful King of the East, Magoa, by my holy labor, by all the names of Divinity, by the name of the All-Powerful; I command thee to obey, and to come to me, or that failing forthwith and immediately to send unto me Massayel, Ariel, Satiel, Arduel Acorib, to respond concerning all that I would know and to fulfill all that I shall command. Else thou shalt come verily in thine own person, to satisfy my will; which refusing, I shall compel thee by all the virtue and power of God.

Conjuration of the King of the South

O Egym, great king of the South, I conjure and invoke thee by the most high and holy names of God, do thou here manifest, clothed with all thy power; come before this circle, or at least send me forthwith Fadal Nastrache, to make answer unto me, and to execute all my wishes. If thou failest, I shall force thee by God Himself.

Conjuration of the King of the West

O Baymon, most potent King, who reignest in the Western quarter, I call and I invoke thee in the name of the Deity! I command thee by virtue of the Most High, to send me immediately before this circle the spirit Passiel Rosus, with all other spirits who are subject unto thee, that the same

*may answer in everything, even as I shall require them. If
thou failest, I will torment thee with the sword of fire
divine; I will multiply thy sufferings and will burn thee.*

Conjuration of the King of the North

*O thou Amaymon, King and Emperor of the Northern
parts, I call invoke, exorcise and conjure thee, by the virtue
and power of the Creator, and by the virtue of virtues, to
send me presently, and without delay, Madael, Laaval,
Bamlahe, Belem and Ramath, with all other spirits of thine
obedience, in comely and human form! In whatsoever place
thou now art, come hither and render that honor which
thou owest to the true living God, Who is thy Creator. In
the name of the Father, of the Son and of the Holy Ghost,
come therefore, and be obedient, in front of this circle,
without peril to my body or soul. Appear in comely human
form, with no terror encompassing thee. I conjure thee
make haste, come straightway and at once!*

[From this point, if more than one participant is involved,
the incantations may be divided up as convenient, although
it may be best if the person who does the invocation of the
four kings also recites the "sacrifice," performs the eucharist, and banishes the forces at the end.]

The Seventh Key

*Rass I Salman Paradiz Oa-Crimi Aao Ial-Pir-Gah Qui-in
Enay Butmon Od I Noas Ni Paradial Casarmg Vgear
Chirlan Od Zonac Luciftan Cors Ta Vaul Zirn Tol Hami
Sobol Ondoh Od Miam Chis Ta Zo Od Es V-Ma-Dea Od
Pi-Bliar O Phil rit Od Miam C-Crimi Quaada. Od. O-
Michaloz Oriom Bagle Papnor I Dlugam Lonshi Od Umplif
V-Ge-Gi Riglied. BABALON!!*

Glory unto the Scarlet Woman, Babylon the Mother of
Abominations, that rideth upon the Beast, for she hath spilt

their blood in every corner of the earth, and lo! she hath mingled it in the cup of her whoredom.

With the breath of her kisses hath she fermented it, and it hath become the wine of the Sacrament, the wine of the Sabbath; and in the Holy Assembly hath she poured it out for her worshippers, and they have become drunken thereon, so that face to face have they beheld my Father. Thus are they made worthy to become partakers of the mystery of this holy vessel, for the blood is the life. So sitteth she from age to age, and the righteous are never weary of her kisses, and by her murders, she seduceth the world. Therein is manifested the glory of my Father, who is truth.

This is the Mystery of Babylon, the Mother of abominations, and this is the mystery of her adulteries, for she hath yielded up herself to everything that liveth, and hath become a partaker in its mystery. And because she hath make herself the servant of each, therefore is she become the mistress of all. Not as yet canst thou comprehend her glory.

Beautiful art thou, O Babylon, and desirable, for thou hast given thyself to everything that liveth, and thy weakness hath subdued their strength. For in that union thou didst *understand.* Therefore art thou called Understanding, O Babylon, Lady of the Night!

O Babylon, Babylon, thou mighty Mother, that rides upon the crowned beast, let me be drunken upon the wine of thy fornications; let thy kisses wanton me unto death, that even I, thy cup-bearer, may *understand.*

And the angel sayeth: Blessed are the saints, that their blood is mingled in the cup, and can never be separate any more. For Babylon the Beautiful, the Mother of abominations, hath sworn by her holy cteis, whereof every point is a pang, that she will not rest from her adultcries until the blood of everything that liveth is gathered therein, and the wine thereof laid up and matured and consecrated, and worthy to gladden the heart of my Father. For my Father is weary with the stress of eld, and cometh not to her bed. Yet shall this perfect wine be the quintessence, and the elixir, and by the draught thereof shall he renew his youth; and so shall it be eternally, as age by age the worlds do dissolve and change, and the universe unfoldeth itself as a Rose, and shutteth itself up as the Cross that is bent into the cube.

And this is the comedy of Pan, that is played at night in the thick forest. And this is the mystery of Dionysus Zagreus, that is celebrated upon the holy mountain of Kithairon. And this is the secret of the brothers of the Rosy Cross; and this is the heart of the ritual that is accomplished in the Vault of the adepts that is hidden in the Mountain of the Caverns, even the Holy Mountain Abiegnus.

And this is the meaning of the Supper of the Passover, the spilling of the blood of the Lamb being a ritual of the Dark Brothers, for they have sealed up the Pylon with blood, lest the Angel of Death should enter therein. Thus do they shut themselves off from the company of the saints. Thus do they keep themselves from compassion and from understanding. Accursed are they, for they shut up their blood in their heart.

They keep themselves from the kisses of my Mother Babylon and in their lonely fortresses they pray to the false moon. And they bind themselves together with an oath, and with a great curse. And of their malice they conspire together, and they have power, and mastery, and in their cauldrons do they brew the harsh wine of delusion, mingled with the poison of their selfishness

The Key of the Thirty Aires (rendered in English)

O you hevens which dwell in ZOM, are mighty in the parts of the Earth, and execute the Judgment of the highest: to you it is said, Behold the face of your God, the beginning of comfort; whose eyes are the brightness of the hevens which provided you for the government of the earth, and her unspeakable variety furnishing you with a power of understanding to dispose all things according to the providence of he that sitteth on the Holy Throne and rose up in the beginning, saying: The Earth, let her be governed by her parts and let there be Division in her, that the glory of her may be always drunken and vexed in itself. Her course, let it run with the hevens; and as a handmayd let her serve them.

One season, let it confound another; And let there be no creature upon or within her the same.

All her members, let them differ in their qualities: And let there be no one Creature equal with another:

The reasonable creatures of the Earth let them vex and weed out one another:

And the dwelling places let them forget their names.

The work of man, and his pomp, let them be defaced, his buildings let them become caves for the beasts of the field.

Confound her understanding with darkness. For why?

It repenteth me I made man, One while let her be known, and another while a stranger;

Because she is the bed of a Harlot, and the dwelling place of him that is fallen!

O you heavens, arise, the lower heavens underneath you, let them serve you;

Govern those that govern

Cast down such as fall

Bring forth with those that increase, and destroy the rotten!

No place let it remain in one number. Add and Diminish, until the stars be numbered:

ARISE, MOVE, and APPEAR before the Covenant of his mouth, which he hath sworn unto us in his Justice.

OPEN the mysteries of your creation

And Make Us Partakers Of Undefiled Knowledge!!!

[The celebrant prepares and gives offering]:

For the forces and beings called upon by this ritual, we give, to feed your power and give you entrance to our world.

Accept this, and honor us by walking among us tonight.

Te Adore, Et Te Invoco!

[Offering made.]

Blackness, blackness intolerable, before the beginning of the light. This is the first verse of Genesis. Holy art thou Chaos, Chaos, eternity, all contradictions in terms!

Oh blue! Blue! whose reflection in the Abyss is called the Great One of the Night of Time; between ye vibrateth the Lord of the Forces of Matter.

O Nox, Nox, qui celas infamiam infandi nefandi, Deio solo sit laus qui dedit signum non scribendum. Laus virgini cuius stuprum tradit salutem.

O Night, that givest suck from thy paps to sorcery, and theft, and rape and gluttony, and murder, and tyranny, and to the nameless Horror, cover us, cover us, cover us from the rod of Destiny; for Cosmos must come, and the balance be set up where there was no need of balance, because there was no injustice, but only truth. But when the balances are equal, scale matched with scale, then will Chaos return.

O thou that hast beheld the City of the Pyramids, how shouldst thou behold the House of the Juggler? For he is wisdom and wisdom hath he made the Worlds, and from that wisdom issue judgments 70 by 4, that are the 4 eyes of the double-headed one; that are the 4 devils, Satan, Lucifer, Leviathan, Belial, that are the great princes of the evil of the world.

And Satan is worshipped by men under the name of Jesus; and Lucifer is worshipped by men under the name of Brahma; and Leviathan is worshipped by men under the name of Allah; and Belial is worshipped by men under the name of Buddha.

And for this is Babalon under the power of the magician, that she hath submitted herself unto the work; and she guardeth the Abyss. And in her is a perfect purity of that which is above; yet she is sent as the redeemer to them that are below. For there is no other way into the supernal mystery except through her, and the beast on which she rideth; and the Magician is set beyond her to deceive the brothers of blackness, lest they should make unto themselves a crown; for if there were two crowns then should Ygdrasil, that ancient tree, be cast out into the Abyss, uprooted and cast down into the Outermost Abyss, and the Arcanum which is in the Adytum should be profaned; and the Ark should be touched, and the lodge spied upon by them that are not masters, and the bread of the Sacrament should be the dung of Choronzon; and the wine of the sacrament should be the water of Choronzon; and the incense should be dispersion; and fire upon the Altar should be hate. But lift up thyself; stand, play the man, for behold! there shall be revealed unto thee the Great Terror, the thing of awe that hath no name.

And this is the mystery that I declare unto thee: that from the Crown itself spring the three great delusions; Aleph is madness, and Beth is falsehood and Gimel is glamour. And these three be greater than all, for they are beyond the words that I speak unto thee; how much more therefore are they beyond the words that thou transmittest unto men.

Behold! the Veil of the Aethyr sundereth and is torn like a sail by the breath of the tempest, and thou shalt see him as from afar off. This is that which is written, "Confound her understanding with darkness," for thou canst not speak this thing.

It is the figure of the Magus of the Taro; in his right arm the torch of the flames blazing upwards; in his left the cup of poison, a cataract into Hell. And upon his head the evil talisman, blasphemy and blasphemy and blasphemy, in the form of a circle. That is the greatest blasphemy of all." On his feet has he the scythes and swords and sickles; daggers; knives; every sharp thing—a million-fold and all in one. And before him is the Table that is a Table of wickedness, the 42-fold table. This Table is connected with the 42 assessors of the Dead, for they are the Accusers, whom the soul must baffle; and with the 42-fold name of God, for this is the mystery of Iniquity, that there was ever a beginning at all. And this Magus casteth forth, by the might of his four weapons veil after veil; a thousand shining colors, ripping and tearing the aethyr, so that it is like jagged saws, or like broken teeth in the face of a young girl, or like disruption, or madness. There is a horrible grinding sound, maddening. This is the mill in which the Universal Substance, which is ether, was ground down into matter.

[The celebrant bows before altar or image and says]:

Deus, tu conversus vivificabis nos. Et plebs tua laetabitur in te. Ostende nobis, Domine, misericordiam tuam. Et salutare tuum da nobis. Domine, exaudi orationem meam. Et clamor meus ad te veniat. Dominus vobiscum. Et cum spiritu tuo.

[Celebrant or another reads]:

And I stood upon the sand of the sea, and saw a beast rise up out of the sea, having seven heads and ten horns, and upon his horns ten crowns, and upon his heads the name of blasphemy.
And the beast which I saw was like unto a leopard, and his feet were as the feet of a bear, and his mouth as the mouth of a lion; and the dragon gave him his power, and his seat, and great authority.
And I saw one of his heads as it were wounded to death; and his deadly wound was healed; and all the world wondered after the beast.

And they worshipped the dragon which gave power unto the beast; and they worshipped the beast, saying

Quis Similis Besteia? Et Quis Poterit Pugnare Cum Ea?

(Who is like unto the Beast? And who can make war with him?)

And there was given unto him a mouth speaking great things and blasphemies; and power was given unto him to continue forty and two months.

And he opened his mouth in blasphemy against God, to blaspheme his name, and his tabernacle, and them that dwell in heaven.

And it was given unto him to make war with the saints, and to overcome them; and power was given him over all kindreds, and tongues and nations.

And all that dwell upon the earth shall worship him, whose names are not written in the book of life of the Lamb slain from the foundation of the world.

If any man have an ear, let him hear.

He that leadeth into captivity shall go into captivity; he that killeth with the sword must be killed with the sword. Here is the patience and the faith of the saints.

And I beheld another beast coming up out of the earth; and he had two horns like a lamb, and he spake as a dragon.

And he exerciseth all the power of the first beast before him, and causeth the earth and them which dwell therein to worship the first beast, whose deadly wound was healed.

And he doeth great wonders, so that he maketh fire come down from heaven on the earth in the sight of men.

And deceiveth them that dwell on the earth by the means of those miracles which he had power to do in the sight of the beast; saying to them that dwell on the earth, that they should make an image to the beast, which had the wound by a sword and did live.

And he had power to give life unto the image of the beast, that the image of the beast should both speak and cause that as many as would not worship the image of the beast should be killed.

And he causeth all, both small and great, rich and poor, free and bond, to receive a mark in their right hand, or in their foreheads:

And that no man might buy or sell save he that had the mark, or the name of the beast, or the number of his name.

Here is wisdom. Let him that hath understanding count the number of the beast; for it is the number of a man; and his number is SIX HUNDRED, THREE SCORE, AND SIX.

[The celebrant makes a chalice and paten (with a form of host) available upon the altar and lifting the chalice intones]:

Offerimus tibi, domine, calicem salutaris, tuam deprecantes clementium; ut in conspectu divinae maiestatis tuae, pro nostra et totius mundi salute, cum odore suavitatis ascendat. Amen.

[He makes the sign of the sun (an equal-armed cross) with the chalice. He then takes the host, holds it above the chalice and says]:

Per eundem Dominum nostrum Primum Mobile filium tuum.

[The celebrant, again on his knees before altar or image says]:

My sovereign Savior Animality, emanation of the Prime Mover, thou who for the salvation of all sentience didst suffer birth into the world of cross and crescent, thou who hast vouchsafed to thy faithful the privilege of making daily commemoration thereof; do thou deign unto thine unworthy servant thus holding thy Living Body in his hands, all strength and ability for the profitable application of that power with which we have been entrusted.

[The eucharist is consumed.]

All that is ordered and stable is shaken, The Aeon of Wonders is come. Like locusts shall they gather themselves together the servants of the Star and of the Snake, and they shall eat up everything that is upon the earth. For why? Because the Lord of righteousness delighteth in them.

The prophets shall prophesy monstrous things, and the wizards shall perform monstrous things. The sorceress shall be desired of all men, and the enchanter shall rule the earth.

Blessing unto the name of the Beast, for he hath let loose a mighty flood of fire from his manhood, and from his womanhood hath he let loose a mighty flood of water. Every thought of his mind is as a tempest that uprooteth the great trees of the earth, and shaketh the mountains thereof. And the throne of his spirit is a mighty throne of madness and desolation so that they that look upon it shall cry: Behold the abomination!

Of a single ruby shall that throne be built and it shall be set upon an high mountain, and men shall see it afar off. Then will I gather together my chariots and my horsemen and my ships of war. By sea and land shall my armies and my navies encompass it, and I will encamp round about it, and besiege it, and by the flame thereof shall I be utterly devoured. Many lying spirits have I sent into the world that my Aeon might be established, and they shall all be overthrown.

Great is the Beast that cometh forth like a lion, the servant of the Star and of the Snake. He is the Eternal one; he is the almighty one. Blessed are they upon whom he shall look with favour, for nothing shall stand before his face.

And every mystery that hath not been revealed from the foundation of the world he shall reveal unto his chosen.

And they shall have power over every spirit of the Ether; and of the earth and under the earth; on dry land and in the water; of whirling air and of rushing fire. And they shall have power over all the inhabitants of the earth, and every scourge of God shall be subdued beneath their feet. The angels shall come unto them and walk with them and the great gods of heaven shall be their guests.

[Here, divination, meditation or sexual activity may take place after which the celebrant recites the final oath and banishing]:

I cling unto the burning Aethyr like Lucifer that fell through the Abyss, and by the fury of his flight kindled the air.

And I am Belial, for having seen the Rose upon thy breast, I have denied God.

And I am Satan! I am Satan! I am cast out upon a burning crag!

And the sea boils about the desolation thereof. And already the vultures gather, and feast upon my flesh.

Yea! Before thee all the most holy is profane, O thou desolator of shrines! O thou falsifier of the oracles of truth! Ever as I went, hath it been thus. The truth of the profane was the falsehood of the Neophyte, and the truth of the Neophyte was the falsehood of the Zelator! Again and again the fortress must be battered down! Again and again the pylon must be overthrown! Again and again must the gods be desecrated!

[Banishing]

Ite in pace ad loca vestra, et pax sit inter vos redituri ad mecum vos invocavero.

In nomine patris, et filii, et spiritus sancti, AMEN.